New Evidence for the Dating and Impact of the Black Death in Asia

THE MEDIEVAL GLOBE

The Medieval Globe provides an interdisciplinary forum for scholars of all world areas by focusing on convergence, movement, and interdependence. Contributions to a global understanding of the medieval period (broadly defined) need not encompass the globe in any territorial sense. Rather, *TMG* advances a new theory and praxis of medieval studies by bringing into view phenomena that have been rendered practically or conceptually invisible by anachronistic boundaries, categories, and expectations. *TMG* also broadens discussion of the ways that medieval processes inform the global present and shape visions of the future.

Submissions are invited for future issues: please contact the Editorial Board (medievalglobe@illinois.edu). All articles will be evaluated by the editors and by a double-blind peer review process. For more information about TMG, with further details about submissions and peer review policy, please visit the journal's website: arc-humanities.org/our-series/arc/tmg.

 The mark of *The Medieval Globe* was designed by Matthew Peterson and draws on elements derived from six different medieval world maps.

Executive Editor

Carol Symes, *University of Illinois at Urbana-Champaign*

Editorial Board

James Barrett, *Norwegian University of Science and Technology*
Darlene Brooks Hedstrom, *Brandeis University*
Claudia Brosseder, *University of Illinois at Urbana-Champaign*
Felipe Fernández-Armesto, *University of Notre Dame*
Monica H. Green, *Independent Scholar*
Jocelyn Hendrickson, *University of Alberta*
Robert Hymes, *Columbia University*
Elizabeth Lambourn, *De Montfort University*
Yuen-Gen Liang, *National Taiwan University*
Elizabeth Oyler, *University of Pittsburgh*
Rein Raud, *Tallinn University & Freie Universität Berlin*
D. Fairchild Ruggles, *University of Illinois at Urbana-Champaign*
Julia Verkholantsev, *University of Pennsylvania*
Alicia Walker, *Bryn Mawr College*

Editorial Assistant

Meg Cornell

Volume 8.1

New Evidence for the Dating and Impact of the Black Death in Asia

by

ROBERT HYMES and **MONICA H. GREEN**

Edited by

CAROL SYMES

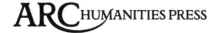

British Library Cataloguing in Publication Data

A catalogue record for this book is available from the British Library.

© **2022, Arc Humanities Press, Leeds**

ISBN (HB): 9781802701012
ISBN (PDF): 9781802701128

www.arc-humanities.org
Printed and bound in the UK (by CPI Group [UK] Ltd).

CONTENTS

LIST OF ILLUSTRATIONS

Charts

Figures

Tables

Plates

Editor's Preface

NEW EVIDENCE FOR THE DATING AND IMPACT OF THE BLACK DEATH IN ASIA

CAROL SYMES

SINCE 2014, WHEN *The Medieval Globe*'s inaugural double issue presented the latest interdisciplinary scholarship on the Black Death, the pace of research on the First (Justinianic) and Second Plague Pandemics has only intensified – alongside the development of new methods for extracting evidence of plague and other diseases from the archaeological, genomic, and documentary records. This special issue brings *TMG* once again to the cutting edge of Black Death studies, featuring a pair of companion articles by leading scholars who contributed to that original issue. And since they have both become members of this journal's Editorial Board in recent years, I want to emphasize that each article has undergone the same rigorous, double-blind peer review process that we observe for all submissions.

The first article is a monumental contribution by Robert Hymes, who presents the fruits of an intensive research project designed to substantiate the hypothesis he offered in 2014. Based on a meticulous survey and analysis of Chinese medical writings spanning nearly a millennium, Hymes offers proof that physicians were adapting their terminology and treatments to the emergence of a virulent new disease, identifiable as plague, beginning in the 1220s. Moreover, the first documented outbreaks of this disease, characterized by purulent lumps or sores, can be linked to the Mongol conquest of North China and a string of sieges, the first three documented between 1213 and 1222. This compelling evidence, carefully contextualized and very clearly explained for non-specialists, suggests that the Second Plague Pandemic had already struck parts of Central and East Asia over a century before it made its reappearance in the greater Mediterranean region.

The second article is by Monica H. Green, whose scholarly vision and leadership was crucial to the success of that inaugural issue. Green locates Hymes's findings, and their implications, within the broader developments of the past eight years, summarizing the extent of our current knowledge about the timing and expanse of the Black Death, and calling for more concerted interdisciplinary efforts to connect such evidence to the new evolutionary history of plague which is emerging from the combination of phylogenetic and palaeogenetic approaches. She thereby offers a generous and truly global perspective on the state of research, identifying the many methodologies and kinds of evidence that must be collected and integrated in order to write the history of an epidemic disease that, as we now know, has been impacting human societies for five millennia. Not only is such collaborative work imperative for furthering our understanding of past plagues, as Green observes, it would provide a model for the still more urgent types of collaboration that are imperative for confronting the global pandemics of our own time, their causes – exacerbated by anthropogenic climate change – and their potential amelioration.

With respect to the history of disease, as with so many other histories, these complementary contributions exemplify the importance of reckoning with the geographical interconnectivity of the medieval globe and its inhabitants, as well as its temporal connections with more distant pasts and more immediate futures.

BUBOES IN THIRTEENTH-CENTURY CHINA: EVIDENCE FROM CHINESE MEDICAL WRITINGS

ROBERT HYMES[*]

IN PATHBREAKING RECENT work, Monica Green has offered the most plausible and comprehensive account to date of the possible routes and mechanisms of the spread of plague across Eurasia in the thirteenth and fourteenth centuries.[1] Green grounds her arguments in the most recent available information on the present distribution of *Yersinia pestis* strains stemming from before and after the polytomy or "Big Bang" that yielded most surviving strains, as well as on a skillful synthesis of previous historical work. She proposes that the polytomy—the explosive divergence of multiple new strains that bacteriological researchers had previously dated to the late twelfth to fourteenth centuries—originated from the Mongols' conquest of the Qara Khitai state (1131–1218) in 1216–1218 (see Table 2.1).

Today, pre-polytomy strains are found solely in the Tian Shan region of what is now Kyrgyzstan on the western border of China:[2] territory that, from 1124 till the 1218 Mongol

---

In my experience, research needs a village—especially when it takes a long time. The ultimate origin of this article, as of my previous contribution to the inaugural issue of *The Medieval Globe*, was Monica Green's invitation in 2014 to join that project by returning to plague in China, on which I had worked briefly but (having no digital databases to exploit at that time) largely inconclusively in the late 1990s. Green's intellectual companionship, advice, and work have been constantly important to me since then as I have pursued further inquiries into plague in middle-period China. Stephen Boyanton, my doctoral student, author of a superb dissertation on the history of literati medicine and "Cold Damage" studies in the Song dynasty, now an independent scholar doing important work in Chinese medical history, and a practitioner of Chinese medicine himself, has repeatedly been an authoritative guide to Chinese medicine; he was also the first to call my attention, at around the same time as Green's invitation, to Li Gao's work treated here. Marta Hanson read earlier versions of this article and was both an encouraging and a useful critic. Hannah Barker was kind enough to share a pre-publication version of her article cited here. Nukhet Varlık gave me a preview of more than one contribution to her forthcoming co-edited volume on death and disease. Conversations with Timothy Brook were helpful at an early stage, as his work has been useful to me since. From the beginning, conversation and exchange of ideas with my son Saul Hymes, a physician specializing in infectious disease, have been intellectually stimulating and, because of who he is, personally precious to me. Along the way Ilana Harwayne-Gidansky, a physician specializing in intensive care, has shown me how manifoldly valuable a daughter-in-law can be by contributing medical expertise of her own. Finally, Carol Symes has been a patient, sympathetic, and careful editor and source of advice in guiding the article to publication. My heartfelt thanks go to all.

1 Green, "The Four Black Deaths" (2020).

2 While this article was already in the production, the new *Nature* report by Spyrou et al., "Source of the Black Death" (2022), was released. The piece is important and welcome in confirming definitively from ancient-DNA (aDNA) evidence what many had long suspected: that the burials at Issyk Kul, which were already known to date from an epidemic year in 1338–1339, represent deaths from plague. Their findings also reinforce Green's suggestion of the Tian Shan region as the site of the plague polytomy or "Big Bang"—previously established in Cui et al., "Historical Variations"

conquest, lay within the Qara Khitai ("Black Khitan") state, also known as Western Liao, founded by Khitan people who had fled the Jurchen conquest of their original Liao state (907–1125) to the east. Green argues that the Mongols' conquest of Qara Khitai brought them into first contact with the bacillus there, whence their own movements carried it to other parts of Eurasia, while shipments of grain ultimately brought it within reach of Europe.

Table 2.1. States and Notable Persons.

States (governed both north and south China, unless otherwise specified)	Dates and location
Tang	618–906
Five Dynasties	906–960
Song	960–1127 in north and south China, 1127–1279 only in south China
Xia (Tangut)	1038–1227 in northwest China
Jin (Jurchen)	1127–1234 in north China
Qara Khitai or Western Liao (Khitan)	1131–1218, centred in modern Kyrgyzstan
Yuan (Mongols)	1234–1279 only in north China, 1279–1369 in north and south China
Ming	1369–1644
Qing (Manchus)	1644–1911
Li Gao	(1180–1251), physician and witness at siege of Kaifeng, 1232–1233
Yuan Haowen	(1190–1257), Jin officeholder and writer

Green has generously treated my previous work as foundational for the view that plague was already in China in the early decades of the thirteenth century and was associated with Mongol sieges in multiple cities in North China under the Jin state.[3] She notes the

---

(2013)—since the graves in which these plague victims were originally buried lie within that region. However, the piece also asserts a late date for the polytomy that, in my view and the view of other historians including Green, is not well supported by their genetic findings. We know that the pre-polytomy strains that survive to this day in that region are fairly little changed: only fifteen or so new SNPs (Single Nucleotide Plymorphisms) across a span of what must be seven or eight hundred years. From this example it is anything but surprising that the strain they have isolated from the 1338 victims should also have changed little since its origin, and this fact itself certainly does not exclude the possibility that the polytomy, wherever it occurred, could have happened more than a century earlier, which Green's work makes still likely. Yet the argument I make here does not depend on any particular date or place for the polytomy, as the plague bacilli that the Mongols brought with them into north China might very possibly have been pre-polytomy strains developed earlier in the bacillus's lineage than the strain Spyrou et al. have isolated; and the polytomy may have followed— very probably stage by stage and one diverging line at a time, rather than all in a single historical moment—as the Mongols made their way back and forth across Eurasia in the decades that followed and as presumably the bacillus found new host species in new environments.

3 Hymes, "Epilogue: A Hypothesis" (2014).

provocative coincidence of patterns in my findings for China with what is now known about plague in Western Asia: that outbreaks were not simply associated with Mongol sieges but began after the sieges were *lifted*.[4] In my own view, my previous work had not placed its claim on a firm enough foundation, but simply framed a hypothesis. On the one hand more positive evidence was needed, while on the other hand a glaring historiographic issue remained largely unaddressed: if the Black Death was in China before it was in Europe, why don't we already know? Why was it not the cataclysm in China's historiography that it was in Europe's? In the present study, I seek to provide a foundation in firmer evidence, drawn largely from thirteenth- through seventeenth-century Chinese medical texts, and at the same time to offer a partial answer, in the specific arena of medical sources, to the question of historiographic near-silence. Larger answers to that historiographic question may be available, I think, in deeper study of the nature of Chinese sources in comparison to those surviving from medieval Europe, and I hope to explore such further answers in future work; but I offer some tentative suggestions in that direction in my conclusion. For now, I hope the present work provides a solider and more precisely shaped puzzle-piece for the puzzle Green has tentatively assembled.

Green's picture of a polytomy set off by the Mongol conquest of Qara Khitai differs significantly, as she notes, from the proposal I had put forth in my previous work: that the key initial contact of the Mongols with *Y. pestis* occurred in their conquest of the Xia state of the Tangut people, in what is now China's Gansu province, a conquest that began with mere raids in 1206 and 1211 but that culminated in the Xia state's total destruction in a devastating campaign spanning 1226 and 1227. At the time of that study, the most recent work on *Y. pestis*'s likely history, based on collection of bacillus strains and their genetic analysis, had concluded that the epicentre of the polytomy was probably the Qinghai Lake region in northeastern Tibet,[5] which lies cheek by jowl with the Gansu corridor and with the intervening mountain range along the other side of which one of the two Mongol armies marched in 1225–1227. Thus my suggested picture fitted well with what we knew about the bacillus then—which was less than we know now.

Green's new Kyrgyzstan-focused picture is based on more recent and much broader knowledge of the bacillus's current distribution, and on that basis is highly plausible. However, nothing in the present article depends on whether it was the Xia conquest or the Qara Khitai conquest that first put the Mongols in touch with the plague bacillus; the most important findings I offer here are largely consistent with either view. I retain, though, some sense that there may be reasons to continue to entertain the Xia hypothesis (or other possibilities as yet unsuggested), and in the afterword to this article I will return to this question. The more basic question the article seeks to answer is: Why, based on Chinese testimony, should we think that the plague was in China at the time of the Mongol conquest at all? Do we have strong enough reason to believe that the Black Death had an East Asian phase?

---

4 Green, "The Four Black Deaths" (2020), 1621. See also Fancy and Green, "Plague and the Fall of Baghdad" (2021).

5 Cui et al., "Historical Variations" (2012).

Preliminary Considerations: Li Gao's Testimony and Problems of Method

In *Plagues and Peoples*, William McNeill was willing to go so far as to claim that the Black Death began in East Asia, though his documentary evidence was minimal and his argument did not find much acceptance among those who studied the Mongols or China.[6] My argument here follows on my previous work (and joins Green's more recent picture) in shifting the earliest phases of the Second Pandemic back by more than a century, but I hope on much stronger evidence than McNeill could adduce. Well after McNeill wrote, both Fan Xingzhun and Cao Shuji (first writing by himself and then in collaboration with Li Yushang) argued for plague in China in the eleventh through thirteenth centuries and beyond.[7] I will draw extensively here on the evidence they used, but will show that, by treating chronology more strictly than they do and thus treating the same sources in a more thoroughly historical way, one unearths a sharp change in the way Chinese medical writings—prescription guides, casebooks, and works of theory—described epidemic diseases.[8] Specifically, in the early-to-middle thirteenth century, a brand new symptom emerged in Chinese epidemic descriptions: a large and purulent sore. This change provides good reason to believe that epidemics fitting the new descriptions and exhibiting the new symptom came into China with the Mongol invasions of the Jin state (1127–1234) of northern China in the early decades of the thirteenth century. Medical writers continued to include these modified epidemic categories and their peculiar new symptom in their compilations on disease and medications through the Mongols' own Yuan dynasty (1234–1369) and the succeeding Ming (1369–1644) and Qing (1644–1911) dynasties, suggesting as well that the new epidemic disease recurred across centuries. The nature and timing of the new descriptions support an identification of the new symptom as the bubo and the new disease as plague.

It appears, from Hannah Barker's recent work, that the old and famous story that the Black Death entered the medieval Mediterranean world via the Mongols' siege of Caffa on the Crimean Peninsula in 1347 is not true: plague probably came to Caffa (whence it would proceed by ship to Europe) by the more mundane channel of grain shipments from various points across the Black Sea.[9] But fully a century before the Caffa siege,

---

6 McNeill, *Plagues and Peoples* (1976), 132–75.

7 Fan, *Zhongguo yishi* shilue (1986), 161–94 and 241-44; Cao and Li, *Shuyi* (2006), especially 60–64. The latter work enlarged greatly upon Cao's earlier article "Dili huanjing" (1995).

8 Fancy and Green similarly use a change in Arabic writings on plague, after the Mongol conquest of Baghdad in 1258, as evidence that that conquest was accompanied by an outbreak of plague: "Plague and the Fall of Baghdad" (2021). The case in China is somewhat different, since in western Asia there was a previous medical awareness of plague as a specific entity, dating back to the Justinianic Plague of the sixth century CE; but the parallel fact of change in medical descriptions after a new encounter with disease is still striking. The same change is explored in greater depth by Fancy, "Knowing the Signs" (2022).

9 Barker, "Laying the Corpses" (2021). For the older story, see for example Horrox, ed., *The Black Death* (1994), 14ff. Fancy and Green, meanwhile, have firmly documented a different case of plague

a medical author recounted a devastating epidemic he had witnessed after a Mongol army lifted its siege of a different Eurasian city. The Jin dynasty physician Li Gao 李杲 (1180–1251), later to be called founder of the "Internal Damage" (*neishang* 內傷 內傷) theory of Chinese medicine, wrote in 1247 of what he had seen between the phases of the 1232 Mongol siege of the Jin's southern capital Daliang 大梁 (modern Kaifeng, Henan province).

> At the time of the change of eras, in the *renchen* 壬辰 year [1232], the capital was at maximum readiness by the second ten days of the third month [May 4 to 14].[10] In all it had been half a month since contact with the enemy, and after the siege was lifted,[11] all but one or two out of every ten thousand people of the capital became sick, and among the sick those who died followed one another without end. At each of the capital's twelve gates, [the dead] sent out each day were two thousand at most and no less than one thousand at fewest, and this was so for almost [two] months. [...]Further back, during the Zhenyou and Xingding eras [1213–1222], [cities] like Dongping, like Taiyuan, or like Fengxiang were all the same in the illness and death they suffered after their sieges were lifted.[12]

In other work, I have shown that the poet and statesman Yuan Haowen supports Li Gao's testimony on two of the siege cities, Taiyuan and Fengxiang, which are mentioned (in passing) in a pair of epitaphs that praise their subjects (each of whom held office near the respective city in years that correspond to temporary Mongol sieges there) for their success in coping with (unspecified) epidemics in the region. The siege years that Yuan's epitaphs indirectly indicate are 1216 for Taiyuan and 1222–1223 for Fengxiang, while Dongping (not mentioned by Yuan) fell under Mongol siege in 1225.[13]

It is important to notice that Li is describing *multiple* epidemic outbreaks of comparable mortality to the Kaifeng (Daliang) episode of 1232, spread across most of North China over a time span of ten years—or seventeen when we count Kaifeng itself—and all associated with Mongol sieges. Through his repeated use of the preposition "like" (*ru* 如)—"like Dongping, like Taiyuan, or like Fengxiang," he is clearly implying that the three episodes he troubles to name were not the only siege-related epidemics of such form and magnitude. That is, he is testifying to a *pattern* of siege-related epidemics ranging across North China and across two decades. I have also shown that Li Gao was well

---

closely associated with a Mongol siege, that of Baghdad in 1258. Their finding strengthens my confidence in Li Gao's account of such an association in multiple north Chinese cities forty-odd to twenty-six years earlier, and also strengthens the case that the epidemic disease in these Chinese cases was also plague.

10 According to the official history of the Jin, the siege had begun on April 28: see *Jinshi*, 17:386.

11 The siege was lifted on May 8 according to the official history: *Jinshi*, 17:387.

12 Li Gao, *Nei wai shang bian huo lun*, 8–9. All translations are my own unless otherwise indicated. The Chinese text has "for almost three months." I have emended this to "almost two months" because the official Jin history and other testimony make the period of the epidemic fifty to sixty days. The Chinese character for three (三) is very similar to the character for two (二), and a scribal or typographical mistake of one for the other, through addition or omission of a single stroke, is not uncommon in premodern Chinese texts.

13 Hymes, "A Tale of Two Sieges" (2021), 302–15.

equipped to have heard about epidemic events in all parts of North China in the relevant years, as his circle of gentlemanly associates and patients included men from all corners of the Jin empire.[14] We know, too, that before the Kaifeng epidemic, Li was particularly renowned as a doctor of febrile and epidemic diseases and of bodily sores: perhaps an ideal combination of specialties for an observer of plague.[15] Yet Li Gao gives us very little physical description of the epidemics he observed at Kaifeng and heard of elsewhere, as he mentions them only in his preface to a work of high and fairly abstract medical theory that (he says) the epidemics spurred him to develop. What he does tell us will be easier to understand after we have first surveyed the evidence of other medical texts.

In arguing that the surviving medical evidence supports an advent of plague within China during the first decades of the thirteenth century, I thus diverge from Cao and Li's proposal, echoing Fan's earlier arguments, that their evidence also demonstrates plague epidemics in the Song (960–1279) and early Jin (1115–1234) dynasties.[16] Although it is important for my argument, too, that epidemic diseases of other kinds were already demographically and culturally important from the Song on, my claim is that the epidemics documented by Li Gao, dating from 1216–1232, constitute the first (known) advent of plague within the cycle of what has become known as the Second Plague Pandemic: the cycle that includes the Black Death in western Asia, Europe, and Africa and that continued via periodic recurrences down through the seventeenth century.[17]

Any historian who proposes that plague devastated cities all across North China in the thirteenth century must confront, again, an obvious question: Why have we not already known this, and for a very long time? Nobody needs to "discover" or "show" that there was demographically disastrous plague in Europe during the fourteenth century; the documentary record is rich, and we have an increasing amount of archaeological and aDNA (ancient DNA) evidence, too. It is clear that if plague had any significant presence in Song-to-Ming China, whatever its demographic impact may have been—and in my view it was large[18]—its historiographic impact was very different than in Europe: in the

---

14 Hymes, "A Tale of Two Sieges" (2021), 316–27; and see also the map of his patients' and associates' places of origin, 326.

15 Yuan Haowen, "Shanghan huiyao yin" 傷寒會要引, in his *Yuan Yishan wenji jiaobu, xia* 下:1272.

16 See Cao and Li, *Shuyi* (2006); Fan Xingzhun, *Zhongguo yishi shilue* (1986).

17 Whether the Tang dynasty epidemics that preceded the Second Pandemic by four to five centuries were plague, as Denis Twitchett argued they might be, and thus perhaps belong to the First Plague Pandemic along with the Justinianic Plague, lies beyond the scope of this article and my larger project: see Twitchett, "Population and Pestilence" (1979). In important and intriguing work, Rodo Pfister has also suggested a Tang and pre-Tang presence and, even more importantly, specific medical awareness of plague in China, embodied in the medical term *ehe zhong* 恶核肿, "evil-kernel swelling," which he treats as possibly referring to plague buboes. It is notable that the term does not appear in the sources I use here, suggesting perhaps that awareness of the term, the symptom it stood for, and the disease—if present in the Tang—had lapsed in between, creating a need that the new application of the term *geda* (see below) could fill. The term had previously been noticed by Wu Lien-teh and others, but Pfister has shown its occurrence in sources previously unnoticed: "Üble Kerne unter der Haut" (2019).

18 On population loss of perhaps forty percent between ca. 1210 and ca. 1290 in North China,

long run, at least, virtually nonexistent. European long-term historical memory, carried in edicts, letters, diaries, chronicles, and eventually in virtually culture-wide general historical awareness, included the memory of an epic catastrophe, subcontinental in span; Chinese long-term historical memory, it seems, did not—or at least not of catastrophic epidemics. This in itself is why many scholars of Chinese history have been deeply skeptical of the notion of "the Black Death in China."

It is easy, I think—perhaps indeed it is an occupational disease—for historians of China to be too confident in the comprehensiveness of our sources. In the present case, while the official history of the Jin does confirm Li Gao's account of the 1232 epidemic at Kaifeng,[19] it is worth pointing out that it is only through Li's own very brief mention, in his preface to just one of his several books, that we have any clear record of the three major epidemic outbreaks *outside* Kaifeng which, if he is right, killed hundreds of thousands or perhaps millions in North China in the second and third decades of the thirteenth century. Further, without Li Gao's clear and specific record, the historian would have little chance of recognizing Yuan Haowen's passing mentions, in two of his many epitaphs, as confirmations. Make this one book disappear, then, and we would know almost nothing. When three disastrous epidemics leave only a single direct record, it is fair to wonder how many others occurred but left none. Whether and to what degree the sources that *do* survive reflect contemporary awareness of a disease that, elsewhere, was both demographically and historiographically devastating—and if not, why not—is a pressing question for the historian. In fact, as I will argue here, the impact of plague *is* reflected in the surviving writings of Chinese medicine—an impact that lasted through the Ming (1368–1644) and into the Qing (1644–1911) dynasty, perhaps renewed through repeated plague encounters.

As noted above, Cao Shuji's 1995 article pointed to plague only at the time of the Mongol conquests and in the subsequent Yuan dynasty. His important 2006 book in collaboration with Li Yushang turned to medical sources he had not previously explored and (like Fan Xingzhun before them) found what they saw as historical attestation of plague epidemics in China a couple of centuries earlier than my thirteenth-century proposal would suggest.[20] In my previous work, I expressed skepticism of Cao and Li's evi-

---

thus spanning the Yuan conquest and potentially even leaving some fifty more years for recovery (suggesting still larger initial loss), see note 121 below.

19 *Jinshi*, 17:387, lines 9–10; 17:388, lines 1–2; 64:1532–33.

20 Cao and Li, *Shuyi* (2006), 60–61. Cao, in fact, now appears to believe that even very early medical sources, such as the *Basic Questions* (first part of the *Inner Canon of the Yellow Emperor*, dating to the first century BCE), the *Golden Casket* texts of the *Treatise on Cold Damage and Miscellaneous Disorders* (third century CE), and the *Pulse Classic* (third century CE), preserve records of significant Chinese medical awareness of plague. The most recent relevant genetic study places the origin of plague between 4000 and 7000 years ago based on remains from the Samara region in present-day western Russia. (See Spyrou et al., "Analysis of 3800-Year-Old *Yersinia pestis* Genomes" (2018).) If it was present in eastern Eurasia that early, it is certainly possible or even likely that the Chinese first encountered it very long ago; but that "Cold Damage" disorders simply were (or were sometimes) plague in the third century or earlier, an idea Cao appears to entertain, or that "at this historical stage, plague seems to have been a commonly-seen illness" does not at

dence that pre-Mongol epidemics in Song and Jin were plague,[21] but proper chronological sorting out of their sources, along with others that my own further explorations led me to, had to await further work. This is what I present here.

Some methodological or theoretical assumptions are worth explaining. Cao and Li, as well as Fan, are largely engaged in retrospective diagnosis by matching symptoms: they read descriptions of disease in medical (and a few non-medical) sources of Song, Jin, Yuan, or later date and conclude that the described symptoms match modern understandings of the symptoms of plague. Symptom-matching and retrospective diagnosis have not earned a good name in the recent discourse of the history of medicine, in China or elsewhere.[22] The move to treat historical medical and disease categories in their own terms, as locally and temporally bounded social constructions, has been salutary and in many cases has shifted the field in intellectually more responsible directions. In considering most questions of Chinese medical history, I have no difficulty taking a historicist (or what Marta Hanson calls "historical-conceptual") view. To ask whether, say, a particular Song-dynasty patient who was diagnosed as suffering from "Cold Damage Disorder" (*shanghan bing* 傷寒病) was "really" a victim of (say) diphtheria has as little use, for most historical purposes, as to ask whether a modern American patient with "diphtheria" (and with no contact with Chinese practitioners or concepts) is "really" suffering from Cold Damage Disorder. A "yes" answer will not explain how doctors treated either patient, how the community and society around him reacted to his sickness, how the patient viewed himself—very possibly including his perceptions of his own symptoms—and it is often difficult to see exactly what specific historical payoff it can carry, in the face of all these explanatory failures. Nor is it clear why the two cases should be treated as exclusive alternatives rather than equally possible (or, today, even combinable) constructions of patients', doctors', and others' experiences. From the perspective of the history of Chinese medicine, and indeed for most questions of the history of disease in China, the "biography of disease" model adopted by Marta Hanson, which gives "not only *attention to changes in a disease concept*, but [...] attention to patients as sufferers and practitioners as mediators attempting to alleviate this suffering *to the best of their ability and knowledge in their time*" (emphasis mine), has clear advantages.[23] Such an approach will not give priority or decisive weight to modern biomedical disease categories, and if it attends to them will treat them as evolving and thus "biographicable" historical objects as well. It will write

---

this point strike me as plausible. In any case, this argument lies well beyond the scope of this article or my project.

21 Hymes, "Epilogue: A Hypothesis" (2014), 211–12 ("Afternote").

22 For an excellent statement of the pitfalls of retrospective diagnosis and the value of approaching Chinese disease concepts on their own terms, see Hanson's *Speaking of Epidemics* (2011), 8–11. More recently see her excellent pair of essays on "Late Imperial Epidemiology" (2021), in which she traces an arc in the historiography of disease in China in which a "natural-realist" approach, often centred on retrospective diagnosis, was to a considerable degree superseded by a "historical-conceptual" approach that put historical actors' own categories to the forefront; but she is encouraged by a recent tendency toward a synthesis of the two, in which some scholars have tempered a natural-realist approach with historical-conceptual understandings and methods.

23 Hanson, *Speaking of Epidemics* (2011), 9.

the history of a particular time and place with an eye first to the concepts available, and in many respects determinative, at that time and place.

And yet. As Piers Mitchell has suggested, a bacillus may have a history too—a history that will only be partly about what humans have made of it.[24] If one's question is the possible historical travel of disease far across the boundaries of societies, cultures, and languages—unless one simply rules such questions out of bounds *a priori*[25]—then a need surely arises for bridging concepts which, in principle, cannot be those of any single one of the potentially quite different cultural or medical communities involved or affected at the time. It must be possible for a historian to ask whether a *common object* has been socially or culturally constructed in different ways by people in different places, using different social and cultural construction kits, even while the same historian cares about those constructions and allows that they may well in turn have created non-common cultural objects with, potentially, their own respective local effects.

My argument is that there was such a common object, which societies at both the western and the eastern ends of Eurasia encountered, and of which they were compelled to devise separate constructions in the thirteenth and fourteenth centuries, registering its devastating effect at the western end and possibly grappling with effects still to be investigated at the eastern end. And for want of a better bridging concept, I posit that the common object was the disease which we currently construct as plague. This is, yes, to assume a modern biomedical concept and, from one point of view, to impose it upon the histories of cultural communities none of which (including those in Europe) had the current concept available. But it need not only impose: in the long run, the biomedical concept, too, need not be an unchangeable given. There is no reason why we cannot learn things from a thirteenth- and fourteenth-century Chinese encounter that may change the modern biomedical plague concept, by changing our understanding of the different forms it may take and the different effects it may have in different times or places. Indeed, the current biomedical understanding of plague has changed considerably since the time of its first construction in the late nineteenth and early twentieth

---

24 Mitchell, "Retrospective Diagnosis" (2011), especially 86: "if we want to use that diagnosis to understand the micro-organism causing that disease, how it was spread around the world, and whom it chose to infect, then making a modern biological diagnosis is not only reasonable, but is a key part of the research process."

25 An influential article by Andrew Cunningham can be read precisely as ruling this question out of bounds, by arguing that what physicians today call "plague" is simply not the same entity as what was called "plague" before Alexandre Yersin's isolation of the *Yersinia pestis* bacillus in 1894, and therefore cannot be discussed in relation to it, since the redefinition of plague as the disease caused by the bacillus transformed its identity, rendering it incommensurable with any previous disease concept—including the concept of "plague" that Yersin had in mind when he entered the hut he used for a laboratory and in which he discovered the bacillus: Cunningham, "Transforming Plague" (1992). I am constitutionally suspicious of *a priori* answers to what at least *look* like empirical questions, and elsewhere I have tried to show that Cunningham's notion of an utter transformation of plague's identity is based on a faulty (because too unitary) notion of the conceptualization of disease at any point in time (before or after Yersin's moment), and that it is easy to show continuities of the plague concept pre-Yersin and post-Yersin: see Hymes, "Continuous Transformation?" (2016).

centuries, in part precisely in response to experience with its manifestations under different circumstances in different parts of the world.[26]

In the enterprise I am about, then, one cannot avoid comparing past reports of symptoms to those now associated with the hypothesized common object—in this case, plague as biomedically understood. Still, my method here will not be simple "symptom-matching." It is very unlikely that we can find in Jin–Yuan Chinese medical accounts something that we will point to and simply say "This is plague"—partly because, if there were such a smoking gun, it would have been identified long ago, probably no later than the nineteenth century; but also precisely because we can't expect differing medical traditions with long methodological and theoretical histories of their own, not to mention different histories of disease experience, to construct closely matching categories upon a new disease encounter. Like Cao and Li, I am interested in reported symptoms; and like them, I am proposing that certain reports of epidemics in Chinese sources reflect encounters with an entity that we moderns have constructed as "plague." But as will be clear from the sources I will explore here, premodern Chinese disease accounts, even by medical practitioners, do not always list symptoms; and when they do, they often give us little reason to think they are attempting to list them exhaustively.[27]

At the risk of overgeneralization, I would say that premodern Chinese medical authorities are more concerned with identifying underlying processes than with superficial symptoms, which in their view are not necessarily defining of underlying processes. This does not mean that practitioners were unempirical, or failed to observe what was happening in patients or to hear what patients reported. Nor do I think that the symptoms they could observe or register were pre-limited by their theoretical categories.[28] I argue just the opposite: that pre-existing theoretical categories of epidemic disease could quite easily absorb newly observed symptoms. As a broad view of Chinese medical thinking, I would propose—though granting that this view grows partly out of my investigation of this specific topic—that it was quite empirically sensitive, but that its approach to the relation

---

26 Even to speak of plague's "first construction in the late nineteenth and early twentieth centuries" may give too little credit to continuing change and reconstruction. Since the discovery of the bacillus in 1894, the biomedical concept of plague has evolved repeatedly: first through the realization of the role of fleas and then rats and other rodents in its transmission; next by the reduction of that realization to an almost exclusive focus on the "rat flea," *Xenopsylla cheopis*, and on rats as its bearers, from about 1906 on; next by a more recent relaxation of that exclusive focus and a restored awareness of the role of other rodents and non-rodent mammals (along with other fleas) as carriers, and more importantly the possibility of human-to-human transmission via the human flea, *Pulex irritans*; by the discovery of the "blocked-proventriculus" mode of transmission from flea to flea-bearer, but more recently by the discovery that this is not the only mode, and that fleas can transmit before their proventriculus is blocked, with crucial implications for possible speed of spread; and most recently by the reconstruction of the genome of the plague bacillus, which has incorporated into plague's identity a genetic component that Alexandre Yersin certainly never envisioned. Much of this, aside from the genetic stage, is well covered in Royer, "The Blind Men and the Elephant" (2014).

27 My thoughts in this paragraph are particularly strongly influenced by conversations with my former student Stephen Boyanton.

28 Such pre-limitation may have been prevented precisely by the fact that these practitioners did not think symptoms *essentially* defining of disease categories.

between empirical observations, on the one hand, and general categories that had already proven both theoretically and practically useful, on the other, was often strongly category-preserving.[29] This sometimes yielded an approach to symptoms that one might—from an outsider's perspective—call additive or incorporative. A doctor who felt that he knew, broadly, what category of illness he was encountering in a particular case, but who met a symptom new to him or new to the literature on that category, could register it as a previously unmentioned (and, since diseases were thought to be fluidly responsive to environmental and temporal conditions, perhaps previously non-occurring) symptom of the already known disease entity, in effect expanding that entity to include it.

In reading the textual products of such processes, my question is thus not quite that of Cao and Li (or Fan): "Are the sources of middle-period China identifying and describing plague?" For the reasons above, I think the literal answer must be: No, they are describing disease encounters in their own terms and using their own categories, whether inherited or (only occasionally) completely new. Rather, my question is: Do disease descriptions across the Song–Jin–Yuan–Ming span, including attention to certain symptoms, change in ways that suggest an encounter with a new phenomenon in the period, and can they support a claim that the new phenomenon was some version of plague as now understood? The answer I offer here, of course, is Yes.[30] I hope that my work here may count as what Marta Hanson has seen as a recent and productive tendency toward the combination of "natural-realist" with "historical-conceptual" approaches, taking historical actors' categories seriously and studying their evolution while still drawing on current biomedical conceptions to see what can result from relating the two to one another.[31]

The Evidence

Cao Shuji and Li Yushang, as stated above, argue that certain epidemics of the Song and early Jin were plague.[32] In this, as well as in tracing plague in epidemic records onward through the Yuan dynasty, they ally themselves with Fan Xingzhun's 1986 work and draw extensively on his sources, also bringing sources of their own to bear. Fan, Cao, and Li specifically detect plague in Song–Jin–Yuan outbreaks that the sources refer to as *datou* 大頭, literally "Big Head," or *datou tianxing* 大頭天行, "Big-Head Heaven-Current;" as *leitou* 雷頭, "Thunder Head;" as *shiyi* 時疫, "Seasonal Epidemic," or in particular *shiyi geda*

---

29 Of course there is nothing specifically "Chinese" about this: the conservatism of modern scientists about theoretical categories in the face of superficially contradictory or previously unfamiliar empirical data is well known, and some such urge to preserve categories is probably essential to any productive system of knowledge.

30 When I indicate in this paper that a particular occurrence of a certain disease term is the earliest I have found, or that X number of such mentions occurs across a certain period, I am relying on the Airusheng *Zhongguo jiben guji ku* 中國基本古籍庫 electronic database and the electronic *Siku quanshu* 四庫全書 database (*Wenyuange Siku quanshu dianziban*). Together, these contain a very substantial proportion of surviving Song, Jin, Yuan, and Ming medical works.

31 Hanson, "Late Imperial Epidemiology, Part 2" (2021).

32 Cao and Li, *Shuyi* (2006), especially 60–65.

時疫疙瘩, "Seasonal-Epidemic Lumps/Sores"; as *shidu* 時毒 "Seasonal Toxin"; and, in at least one case, simply as *houbi* 喉閉, "Throat-Closure." In sorting out epidemic descriptions, however, Cao and Li in particular are not strict about the chronology of sources. To my eye, the effect is to conflate across time a variety of sources and disease names and conclude that all represent (in modern biomedical terms) a single disease, from their first mention to the last. I will argue, instead, that certain disease names or categories, which I see no reason to think referred to plague in their first use, later changed by incorporating a symptom unmentioned earlier; and that the change's timing suggests encounters with (in our terms) a new disease. The symptom is lumps or sores, often specifically noted as purulent, suggesting the most salient symptom of (bubonic) plague. Especially important is the essentially new medical term *geda*, which I will translate provisionally as "lumps/sores," but of which there will be much more to say further on.

For my understanding of the sources used by Fan, Cao, and Li—and of others I have unearthed guided partly by theirs—I have found it crucial to construct a detailed timeline, separately registering events, disease descriptions, and the sources that record them across time. I present that timeline in table form below, as reference material for the discussion that will follow.

Table 2.2 Addition of Lumps/Sores (*Geda*) to Pre-Existing Epidemic Disease Categories (please also see the references in Appendix 2.1).

Item	Date	Epidemic Record or Mention, and Name	Lumps / Sores?	Throat Closure?	Head / Face Swelling?
1	1090	Throat Closure (*houbi*) (recorded 1090–1099)	—	+	—
2	1138–1149	[No name]: "presentation similar to Thunder Head (*leitou*)" (recorded 1156–1161)	—	+	+
3	Before 1186	Big Head and Thunder Head Wind (*leitou feng*) (recorded 1186; no dated event mentioned)	—	—	+
4	1202	Seasonal Toxin (*shidu*); Big Head Heaven-Current (*datou tianxing*) (recorded 1266)	—	+	+
	Mongols invade Jin in 1205 and 1206, recurring through the 1210s–1220s until the siege of Kaifeng in 1232 and the fall of Jin 1234				
5	1207–1208	*Nue* (intermittent high fevers) and "miasmic pestilence" (recorded 1228)	+	—	—
6	1213–1222	Unnamed epidemics in Taiyuan, Dongping, and Fengxiang, reported to be similar to that of the 1232 Kaifeng siege epidemic (recorded 1247)	No specifically relevant description	No specifically relevant description	No specifically relevant description

Item	Date	Epidemic Record or Mention, and Name	Lumps / Sores?	Throat Closure?	Head / Face Swelling?
7	Before 1228	Thunder Head (recorded 1228; no dated event mentioned)	+	—	+
8	1232	Kaifeng siege epidemic (recorded 1247): no disease name given, reportedly mistaken for Cold Damage; author proposes reclassifying this and other conditions under new "Internal Damage" category	No specifically relevant description	No specifically relevant description	No specifically relevant description
9	Before 1253	Throat Closure; Big Head; Thunder Head; Seasonal Qi (*shiqi*); Epidemic Qi (*yiqi*) (recorded 1253; no dated event mentioned)	+	+	—
10	Before 1264	Big Head Illness (recorded 1253; no dated event mentioned)	+	—	+
11	Before 1267	Seasonal Toxin; Seasonal Disease (*shiji*) "in presentation similar to Thunder Head" (recorded 1267; no dated event mentioned)	+	+	+
12	Before 1281	Thunder Head Wind ("presenting like Cold Damage") (recorded 1281; no dated event mentioned)	+	—	—
13	Before 1281	Seasonal Toxin (recorded 1281; no dated event mentioned)	+	+	+
14	Before 1281	Seasonal Epidemic (*shiyi*) (recorded 1281; no dated event mentioned)	+	—	—
15	Before 1300? ("Yuan")	Seasonal Epidemic; Swelling Toxin (recorded ~1300; no dated event mentioned)	+	+	+
16	Before 1335	Seasonal Toxin (recorded 1335; no dated event mentioned)	+	+	—
17	Before 1335	Seasonal Toxin; Big Head Illness (recorded 1335; no dated event mentioned)	+	—	—
18	Before 1406	Toxin Swelling; Swelling Toxin (zhongdu); Seasonal Epidemic (recorded 1406; no dated event mentioned)	+	+	+
19	Before 1447	Swelling Toxin; Seasonal Epidemic (no specific event recorded)	+	+	+

As the table's meaning may not be transparent, it is worth summarizing here; a more detailed chronological discussion filling out its implications will follow further on. First, in a series of disease descriptions beginning with an epidemic of 1090 (item 1 above) and comprising sources dating from 1099 on, no explicit mention of purulent lumps or sores is attached to any epidemic before 1207 (item 5); and that 1207 mention is preserved in a source of 1228. It is noteworthy, then, that the first Mongol incursions into the Jin state took place in 1205, and their first full-scale entry into Jin in 1206; that the final conquest of Jin took place in 1234;[33] and that between those dates historical sources mention epidemics among the Mongols or in North China as of 1211;[34] across several cities between 1213 and 1222 (Li Gao's account, item 6); at some time after 1226,[35] and in Kaifeng in 1232 (item 8).

In other words, before the earliest mention of lumps or sores in the extant accounts of epidemic disease contained in the medical sources from 1090 onward (as assembled by Fan, Cao and Li, and myself), the Mongol invasions had intervened, along with a series of epidemics explicitly associated with the Mongols by contemporaries, though for which we do not usually have symptom descriptions. After that earliest 1207/1228 attestation, mention of purulent lumps or sores as characteristic of certain epidemic categories recurs in medical texts of ca. 1253 (item 9), 1264 (item 10), 1267 (item 11), 1281 (three times: item 12, item 13, and item 14) , ca. 1300 (item 15), 1335 (item 16 and item 17), 1406 (item 18), and 1447 (item 19). It is important to notice that four *different* disease terms or categories changed through the addition of the same symptom across this period:[36] "Thunder Head," "Big Head," "Seasonal Toxin," and the much older

---

33 For the Mongol campaigns in and final conquest of Xia, see Wu, *Xi Xia shi gao* (1983), 122–38.

34 In 1211, the chief minister of Jin, arguing for submitting to the Mongols on the theory that they would not stay long in North China, is reported to have said to his ruler, "I have heard that the men and horses of the Tartars [i.e., Mongols], not appropriate to the water and land [in which they find themselves], are experiencing pestilence." Note the clear implication that "pestilence" was not characteristic of the Mongols in their home territories, but had emerged among them on entering territories not their own: see Bao, ed., *Yuanchao mishi* (2005), 173. See also *The Secret History of the Mongols*, ed. and trans. Cleaves (1982), 184 and 186; and the conclusion of this article.

35 In 1226, when the Mongols' Khitan advisor Yelü Chucai (1190–1244) joined in the conquest of two cities in Chinggis Qan's Xia campaign, a later source tells us: "The commanders competed to seize boys, girls, jades, and silks; [Yelü] alone took only several volumes of documents and two camel-loads of rhubarb. Later there was epidemic in the army, and only those who received rhubarb were curable: nearly ten thousand men were saved" (Tao Zongyi, *Chuogeng lu* (1366/1959): chapter 2; quoted in Cao, "Dili huanjing" (1995), 189, with no reference).

36 Note: the great majority of the sources I mine here are general catalogues of diseases or of prescriptions for them; they are mostly *not* historical records of particular disease *events*. Thus I cannot derive, from most of them, a time or place for any particular epidemic outbreak. (The few exceptions in the timeline in which I am dealing with records of particular epidemics are explicitly noted there.) The dates given in the first column, often in the form "Before [year]," thus derive from the dates of authorship or publication of *books*, and are *not* dates of epidemics. My assumption is that if an author describes a disease of a particular kind in a book that he completes or publishes at a particular date, he knows or is under the impression that examples of that disease have actually occurred before that date. It is similarly usually impossible to place the diseases to which such compilations refer in any particular place or region.

and more generic term "Seasonal Epidemic." Each of these will be traced in more detail below.[37] My argument, again, is that all this evidence represents the new appearance, after the Mongol advent in Xia and Jin, of purulent lumps or sores as a symptom added to older epidemic-disease categories that had not previously included them. To show this clearly, it is useful to examine more closely both earlier and later disease descriptions.

Pre-Mongol Epidemic Categories: Closed Throat, Thunder Head, Big Head, and Seasonal Toxin

The most important of the earlier descriptions involve illnesses that, though differently named, all involve obstruction or closing of the throat. Consider Pang Anshi 龐安時 (1032–1099), writing of the 1090 epidemics (item 1 above):

> In the fifth year of the Yuanyou era, from spring through summer and into fall, the people of the two prefectures of Qi and Huang 齊黃 suffered urgent throat-closing (houbi 喉閉). Of every ten [who got it], eight or nine died. In rapid cases they died in half a day or a day. The prefectural judge of Huangzhou, Pan Chengyan 潘昌言, personally lost several members of his lineage. Later he/they obtained Black Dragon Grease, and several dozen were saved.[38]

Compare the testimony of a "Mr. Yang" (Yang shi 楊氏) around 1156 (item 2 above). The later source (ca. 1300) that pastes in a passage attributed to Mr. Yang, as a witness from one hundred and fifty years before (item 15), does so under the heading "Seasonal-Epidemic Lumps/Sores Swelling-Toxin Illness" (shiyi geda zhongdu bing 時疫疙瘩腫毒病). However—and this is crucial—the pasted-in passage itself actually has nothing to say about lumps or sores of any kind:

> Between the Tianjuan [1138–1140] and Huangtong [1141–1149] periods, first north of the ridges,[39] next in Taiyuan 太原, finally in Yan and Ji 燕薊 prefectures, the mountain villages and quarters suffered severely from this affliction, which down to today has not ended. It is transmitted from one [person] to another, in many cases leading to death; there are even those who [when faced with it] do not protect their families. In presentation it is similar to Thunder Head, swelling the throat and neck. If it attacks internally, the throat is blocked, and water and medicine pass with difficulty. If it attacks externally, the head and face are like [those of] an ox, the eye and ear orifices fill up, and looking and listening are both negated, shutting off hearing and seeing. When the illness is serious it endangers life.[40]

---

37 This term, by the way, does not mean that a disease comes in every year with its particular season, or that it is in any sense routine. It refers merely to typical seasonal conditions that *can*, under the right other circumstances (not always well specified or even assumed to be understood), generate a particular disease.

38 Pang Anshi, *Shanghan*, 3:75.

39 *Lingbei* 嶺北. This seems to refer to areas north of Jin territory; in Yuan it will become the name of a province-level unit in Mongolia.

40 "Mr. Yang" 楊氏, *Prescriptions for Rescue and Aid* (*Zhengji fang* 拯濟方), cited in the Yuan collection "Shiyuan's Proper and Effective Prescriptions" (*Shiyuan duanxiao fang* 施圜端效方), quoted in the nineteenth-century Korean compilation *Categorized Collection of Medical Prescriptions* (*Uibang yuch'wi* 醫方類聚), reprinted in China as *Yifang leiju*, 179:419.

We do not know what name, if any, "Mr. Yang" himself had used for this disease, but his description bears striking similarities to the account of an epidemic, in the Jin prefecture of Jiyuan in 1202, that has come down to us from Li Gao through his student Luo Tianyi 羅天益 (item 6). (It is the clear intention of Luo's text that his reader take the account as originating from Li Gao, and I have found no reason to doubt this.) Under the heading "Seasonal Toxin, Treated Effectively" (*shidu zhiyan* 時毒治驗), Luo presents the following narrative:

> In 1202, when my late teacher [i.e., Li Gao], through his donations,[41] was made supervisor of taxes in Jiyuan 濟原, in the fourth month the common people in large numbers were [suffering from] an epidemic disease (*yili* 疫癘). First, they felt abhorrence of cold[42] and heaviness in the body; next it was transmitted to their head and face, which swelled up. Their eyes could not open and they gasped; their throat would not pass [food or drink]; their tongue was dry and mouth parched. It was popularly called "Big Head Heaven-Current." Relatives did not visit each other; if it infected (*ran* 染) them, most were not saved.[43]

Cao and Li, along with Fan Xingzhun before them, seem on strong ground in bringing these three accounts together as separate episodes of a single epidemic disease—especially the latter two. One cannot be sure that all three were placed in the same category by contemporaries on the ground, since Pang Anshi identifies the first simply as "throat-closure," while we do not know what "Mr. Yang" called the 1138–1149 epidemics and Luo Tianyi identifies the 1202 outbreak by its popular name, Big Head. But to see the three as a single new phenomenon that contemporary physicians were striving to name and describe seems reasonable.

Much less obvious is why Fan or Cao and Li see these three earliest of their sources as representing plague. Pang Anshi, for one, gives his description of the 1090 "throat-closing" epidemic in the context of a list of nine different *throat and mouth* ailments, any of which may be treated effectively, as he says that epidemic was, with a certain "Black Dragon" salve, and mentions no other significant symptoms.[44] In fact none of the major symptoms described in any of these accounts—throat-closure, loss of vision or hearing, a general swelling of the head, throat, and neck capable of producing the effect of "a head like an ox"—characterize plague, either currently or (in medieval Christendom and the Islamicate world) historically;[45] and the popular names "Big Head" and "Thun-

---

41 Donations made for famine relief and rewarded with office. See Li Gao's biography in Luo, *Dongyuan shixiao fang*, 9–12.

42 Reading *zenghan* 增寒 as a mistake for homonymous *zenghan* 憎寒. The latter is a standard term for chills.

43 Luo Tianyi, *Dongyuan shixiao fang*, 9:1a.

44 Pang Anshi, *Shanghan*, 3:75.

45 It is far from the object of this study, but nonetheless striking, how reminiscent the symptoms described here are of diphtheria as observed in modernity. Throat blockage (by a pseudo-membrane that grows across the tonsils and larynx) is the standard symptom in severe diphtheria, and the swelling of the throat and neck to match the size of the head may produce an appearance called "bull-neck," which is strikingly parallel to the "head like an ox" mentioned in these sources. I mention this only in passing: it is hard enough to show plague in premodern Chinese sources, and I have no ambition to show diphtheria as well.

der Head" suggest that head-and-neck swelling was, at least originally, by far the most dramatic external symptom to a contemporary non-medical eye. At the same time, the descriptions lack just the symptoms one might expect to be most obvious in outbreaks of plague: either buboes, if the plague were the bubonic form commonly reported in those later Western sources—one looks in vain for any references to lumps or sores in these early Chinese sources—or coughing of blood, if it were the less common but deadlier pneumonic form. The physician Liu Wansu, in 1186, had also described Big Head without any reference to lumps or sores (item 3), mentioning only head-swelling before and behind the ears.[46]

Any impulse to conflate the Big Head disease described by Liu in 1186 and treated by Li Gao in 1202 (as described by Luo Tianyi in 1266) with later outbreaks under that name (which I agree were probably plague) runs up against the crucial fact that Li Gao, in his own 1247 account of the 1232 siege-epidemic in Kaifeng (item 8), *does not* mention any connection or resemblance to the 1202 outbreak that he had treated decades before, much less mention the disease-name "Big Head." Instead he quite assertively connects the 1232 epidemic *only* to other epidemics associated with Mongol sieges in Jin territory between 1213 and 1222 (item 6). Indeed his creation of a new field of medicine—Internal Damage theory—in response to the 1232 epidemic, along with his denial of contemporary physicians' assumption that the culprit disease was Cold Damage disorder (*shanghan* 傷寒), seems to tell us that he understood these epidemics, as a group, to be either unprecedented or never previously recognized. I suspect, in fact, that Fan Xingzhun as well as Cao and Li may identify the earlier epidemics with plague precisely under the influence of the later developments in which purulent lumps begin to be subsumed under the same disease categories.[47] But it is important—and key to my method and argument here—to see that they had *not* yet been so subsumed in these earlier accounts.

Epidemic Categories after the Mongols' Arrival: Adding Lumps or Sores

What of later descriptions? In what follows, I treat the first addition of lumps or sores as newly-specified symptoms to each previously-existing epidemic disease category, one category at a time. Here I am not claiming that *every* mention of lumps or sores compels an inference of buboes and plague. Nor may we assume that every medical authority represented here had actually ever encountered plague—it may be unlikely that they had, since physicians who encountered it might well have died with their patients and left no record of their views. Many doctors whom we read now may describe epidemic diseases they have only heard or read about. What I see in the sources instead is—at

---

46 Liu, *Suwen bingji qiyi baoming ji*, 136–37.

47 See, for instance, Cao's own earlier article arguing for plague at the Ming–Qing transition, "Shuyi liuxing" (1997). "Big Head" disease is prominent in this period as well, and in Cao's argument for plague. Having identified Ming-period Big Head as plague in his 1997 work, I suspect that, in his 2006 book, he then found it natural to identify Jin-period Big Head as plague, as well.

minimum—the spread of a new *idea*, through one disease category after another, that previously-known forms of epidemic disease might display purulent lumps or sores; and my argument is that encounters with plague, after the Mongol incursions, account for the spread of the idea.

The first direct mention of purulent sores in association with epidemic disease in these sources—intriguingly sitting alongside the spitting or coughing of blood—occurs in the *Confucian Service of Kin* (*Rumen shiqin* 儒門事親) of Zhang Congzheng (1156–1228) (item 5), a description that Fan Xingzhun points to as plague. Zhang writes in 1228 of the long-known disease category called *nue* 瘧—characterized by recurrent fever, which accounts for its modern application to malaria (though of course one may not assume that that is what it exclusively labelled in premodern China)—and he mentions epidemics of 1207 and after. He begins with a general discussion of *nue* and its frequent misunderstanding by contemporary doctors, who view it as a manifestation of cold in the spleen, while Zhang understands it as a heat-based disease. Doctors who see it as cold will therefore often treat it with harsh heat-based drugs, in effect piling heat on heat, with disastrous consequences.

> In times of peace and order, usually there is not much *nue*-illness. In times of disturbance and turmoil, often there is much *nue*-illness. In times of peace and order, even if one uses toxic medicines such as arsenic or cinnabar to treat it, one may still obtain a successful result.[48] This is because, in times of peace and order, the people are safe and calm; thus even if one uses heat to attack heat, there will still be few disastrous consequences. But when it comes to times of turmoil, when the people are wearied from toil, one may not abruptly use medications of high toxin or high heat: it is like using heat to attack heat, and when the heat is extreme it will turn into coughing [or vomiting] of blood, passing blood [in urine or faeces], purulent sores [*yongju chuangyang* 癰疽瘡瘍], and vomiting. For in times of turmoil, the ordinances of government are troubled and disordered, drafting of labour is confused and excessive, and with fighting from morning to night there is not the slightest rest. The inner fire and the outer fire are both stirred around, and this is especially severe for those of rank or office. How could they be treated by the same methods as those who are safe and calm? I have personally seen that, in the sixth year of the Taihe period [1206], the South-Campaigning Armies[49] undertook major actions; in the next year [1207], the army returned. That year [still 1207], a miasmic pestilence (*zhangli* 瘴癘) killed I do not know how many people; disorientation and heart-anguish (*aonong* 懊憹) affected eight or nine out of ten. This was all the transformation of fire. The next year [1208], *nue*-illness arose in abundance; those of rank and office all grew ill, in milder cases for a week or month, in more severe cases for a full year.[50]

Stephen Boyanton[51] is certainly right that neither an illness characterized by recurrent fever (the normal application of the term *nue*) nor, all the more, one that lasts a month or

---

48 On the use of medications frankly described as "toxic" or "poisonous" in Chinese medicine, see the excellent recent study by Yan Liu, *Healing with Poisons* (2021).

49 *Zhengnan shilü* 征南師旅. This presumably refers to the Jin counter-incursions into Song at the time of Han Tuozhou's 韓侂胄 anti-Jin war.

50 Zhang Congzheng, *Rumen shiqin*,1:77–78. Stephen Boyanton first called my attention to this passage.

51 Personal communication.

a year for a single patient, can possibly be judged to be plague as now understood; thus this case may be a red herring. But in the first place, Zhang does not tell us that the 1207 outbreak was *nue*; he calls it "a miasmic pestilence," a broader concept with some kinship to *nue* but that, for some reason, he chooses to distinguish from it when he goes on to class the succeeding 1208 outbreak as definitely *nue*. One may wonder what, in the 1207 outbreak, had motivated him to use a vaguer yet potentially more serious term. He seems (though he is not explicit about this) to attribute this epidemic directly to the army's previous sojourn in the south, but he does not tell us why; and for our part we know that in the meantime (in 1205 and 1206) Mongol armies had made incursions into Jin territory.

But whatever Zhang may or may not have seen in the 1207 outbreak, the structure of the text disconnects his discussion of the misidentifications and misprescriptions that lead to a suite of symptoms, including purulent sores and coughing of blood, from the specific account of the epidemics of 1207 to 1208. That is, he does not tell us that he observed the problematic treatments specifically at that time, but rather treats them as issues that *may* occur in cases of *nue* or "miasmic" epidemics in general. Is it possible that, writing in 1228, more than twenty years after the 1207 outbreaks, Zhang has since encountered or heard of epidemic outbreaks characterized by high fever, which he assumed or inferred to be *nue* or "miasmic," but which exhibited coughing of blood and/ or purulent sores and often ended in death; and that he ascribes these symptoms and outcomes to mistaken treatment simply in accord with long-established Chinese medical habit? My larger argument does not depend on Zhang's case, which clearly involves a different disease categorization than any case that follows; but I offer it here as a possibly relevant instance, rather than simply dismissing Fan Xingzhun's view that Zhang is writing of plague.[52]

Epidemic Categories after the Mongols' Arrival: Big Head

Somewhat later than Zhang's account of 1228 is the first direct association of lumps or sores with Big Head. We have seen that, in 1186, Liu Wansu (item 3) had made no mention of them in his discussion of Big Head, mentioning only general head-swelling before and behind the ears. Liu's passage is duplicated verbatim in Li Gao's *Strategic Essentials of the Methods of Life* (*Huofa jiyao* 活法機要), a work of uncertain date but presumably predating Li's own death in 1251:[53] suggesting that Li Gao, who had seen and treated a Big Head epidemic in 1202, later saw nothing to add to Liu Wansu's discussion. But in 1264[54] (item 10), Li's student Wang Haogu 王好古 (traditional dates 1200–1268)

---

52 Fan, *Zhongguo yishi shilue*, 171–72.

53 Li Gao, *Huofa jiyao*, 353–54. Here I join the editors of *Dongyuan yiji* and of *Jin-Yuan si da jia yixue quanshu* in ascribing this work to Li Gao rather than to the Yuan physician Zhu Zhenheng. For a brief but convincing argument of support see *Dongyuan yiji*, introductory matter, 8.

54 The preface to this work is dated "In the Zhida 至大 period [1308–1311], at the change of era, autumn, seventh month, twenty-first day, noted by Wang Haogu formerly of Zhao." The year of the "change of era" to Zhida was 1308; but this conflicts with Wang's traditional dates, ca. 1200–1268. Scholars have resolved the contradiction by assuming "the Zhida period" to be a miswriting of "the Zhiyuan 至元 period" (1264–1294), which would make the year 1264. Since the characters *da* 大

reproduced the same passage verbatim in his transmission of his teacher's ostensible work, entitled *These Matters Are Hard to Know* (*Ci shi nanzhi* 此事難知). It appears under the annotation "below are Li [Gao]'s Twenty-Five Treatises," but with an entirely new passage inserted immediately before the words he had taken (without attribution) from Liu Wansu:

> Now this Big Head Illness,[55] although it is heat-ill that lies in the body and hides in itself, also responds to the four seasons of Heaven and Earth and is fastened upon (*zhu* 著) by unseasonal epidemic *qi*, whereby this disease is produced. It can go so far as to burst so that pus comes out and in turn infects/contaminates other people; for this reason it is called "epidemic."[56]

Thus Liu Wansu's vague head-swelling before and behind the ears has turned into a specifically purulent swelling that can burst and whose pus is infectious. In view of Li Gao's earlier reproduction of the same passage without these added details, it is likely that this addition is Wang Haogu's own. Much later in the same section, but also in a passage of new material found neither in Liu Wansu's description nor in Li Gao's restatement of it, Wang refers more precisely to the possible eruption of *geda*—purulent lumps under the skin.[57] This is the earliest definitely datable occurrence of the term *geda* in epidemic contexts that I have found. Nor was it the only time that Wang mentions *geda* in such contexts: in his *Principal Army of the Fortress of Medicine* (*Yilei yuanrong* 醫壘元戎) (item 9), he prescribes a "Stomach-Regulating Qi-Restraining Decoction" (*tiao wei chengqi tang* 調胃承氣湯), with varying additions, for "Epidemic-Qi, Big Head,[...]Lumps/Sores (*geda*) of Seasonal Qi, Fivefold-Emerging Sores, Throat Closure, and Thunderhead."[58] The date of this work is uncertain; Wang's preface tells us that he had first compiled it in 1237, had lost it (or parts of it) by lending it to an associate, and had recompiled it through long labour after that time. Since there is no reason to think his recompilation duplicated the original, the earliest reliable date for the passage is some significant time after 1237: thus possibly, though not certainly, earlier than the passage in *These Things Are Hard to Know*. In the table above, I provisionally date it to 1253.

---

and *yuan* 元 would be easy to misread for each other in manuscript, I agree that this is the likeliest solution to the conflict; but there remains an outside chance that this work was prefaced in 1308. (This would require either that Wang Haogu's traditional dates are wrong or that the preface is not actually his own.) In that case, 1308 would be the date of the first recorded mention of purulent sores as a symptom of the Big Head illness. This would not essentially affect my argument but would only rearrange the chronology of different authors' incorporation of lumps or sores into the several preexisting categories of epidemic disease I deal with here.

55 "Illness" is my emendation. The original (cited below) has "Big Head Pain" *datou tong* 大頭痛, in which *tong* 痛, "pain," is an easy mistranscription of *bing* 病, "illness," probably facilitated by the commonness of the term *toutong* 頭痛, "headache," in both medical and nonmedical contexts.

56 Wang Haogu/Li Gao, *Cishi nanzhi*, j. *xia*, 77–78. The closing line carries an interesting implication that, for this author and in this context at least, the term "epidemic" (*yi* 疫) inherently entails contagion—by no means a universal view in Chinese medical theory.

57 Wang Haogu/Li Gao, *Cishi nanzhi*, j. *xia*, 79.

58 Wang Haogu, *Yilei yuanrong*, 4:4b.

Epidemic Categories after the Mongols' Arrival: Thunder Head

The passage from Wang Haogu above is the earliest evidence[59] that Thunder Head, like Big Head, has acquired the new symptom. This is echoed somewhat later (ca. 1281) in the work of Li Gao's other student Luo Tianyi (item 12 above). In his *Precious Mirror for Protecting Life* (*Weisheng baojian* 衛生寶鑑), under the rubric "A Prescription for Thunder Head Wind," he offers a "Clearing Invigoration Decoction" specifically to treat "the swelling and pain of lumps/sores" (*geda zhongtong* 疙瘩腫痛) on the head or face, with chills, fever, and with stiffness and tension in the limbs, presenting like Cold Damage."[60]

Post-Mongol Epidemic Categories: Seasonal Toxin and Seasonal Epidemic

In the meantime another medical author, Xu Guozhen 許國禎, had become the first to point out *geda* as a symptom also of Seasonal Toxin (*shidu* 時毒). In his *Prescriptions from the Imperial Hall of Medications* (*Yuyaoyuan fang* 御藥院方), prefaced in 1267, he offered a Seasonal Toxin Medication, which

> treats seasonal disease giving rise to fever, with *geda* in the neck region; chills, high fever, headache, head and face red and swollen, in presentation similar to Thunder Head, and transmitted by contagion from one to another. Those who cannot be saved [by other means] are suited to take this.[61]

"Seasonal Toxin" had been Luo Tuanyi's other name for the epidemics popularly called Big Head and treated by Li Gao in 1202, which Luo had described in 1266 with no mention at all of lumps or sores; but as of 1281, he confirmed Xu Guozhen's new symptomatological picture in another section of his *Precious Mirror* (item 13 above). Here, under the heading "A Prescription for Lumps/Sores [*geda*] of Seasonal Toxin," we read that a *Rhaponticum* Decoction will

> treat accumulated heat in the organs, which manifests itself as swelling-toxin and as the lumps/sores [*geda*] of Seasonal Epidemics (*shiyi* 時疫). The head and face swell, the throat is stopped up, and water and medicine cannot go down. All this is a critical epidemic pestilence (*yili* 疫癘).[62]

---

59 A transitional step may be represented by Zhang Congzheng's note on Thunder Head in 1228, in *Confucian Service of Kin* (item 15 above), which describes "red swelling-cores on the head, sometimes like fresh ginger pieces or jujubes in appearance. One may use a needle to prick them and let out blood: this will forever remove their source." In terms of their described appearance, these could be plague buboes, which can certainly be reddish; but those would probably yield pus more abundantly and noticeably than blood when lanced, which makes one doubt that buboes are what Zhang is talking about or, alternatively, that he has ever actually seen these sores. They do, nonetheless, represent the incorporation of raised and lanceable sores into an epidemic disease category for which these had not previously been described in the sources that survive: Zhang Congzheng, *Rumen shiqin*, 4:330. Marta Hanson (personal communication) has further pointed out that the choice of ginger pieces and jujubes may be intended to indicate a range of possible colours, from pinkish to brownish. It may also be intended to indicate size.

60 Luo Tianyi, *Weisheng baojian*, 9: 371–72. This passage is not cited by Cao and Li or by Fan.

61 Xu Guozhen, *Yuyaoyuan fang*, 7:11a. (*Zhongguo jiben gujiku* citation 7:122.)

62 Luo Tianyi, *Weisheng baojian* 9:373. (Not cited by Fan or by Cao and Li.)

Note that here, more clearly than in any previous example, the most salient symptoms that had once been said to characterize Seasonal Toxin, also called Big Head, in Luo Tianyi's account of Li Gao's 1202 epidemic treatment—generalized head-and-face swelling and throat closure—are carried right over into a new description that incorporates lumps or sores as an additional conspicuous symptom.

In this Luo Tianyi passage, Seasonal Toxin and the much older term Seasonal Epidemic appear as virtual synonyms, or at least as naming the same object. Elsewhere in the same work (item 14), Luo Tianyi uses only Seasonal Epidemic, though still mentioning "toxin," in naming what seems to be the same phenomenon: "Toxin-Dispelling Pill. Treats the ill symptom of *geda* of seasonal epidemic."[63] We will return to Seasonal Epidemic below, but one further example of Seasonal Toxin should come first. Consider the late Yuan physician Qi Dezhi 齊德之, in his *Essential Meanings of the External Specialty* (*Waike jingyi,* dated 1335), under the heading "On Seasonal Toxin" (item 16):

> This Seasonal Toxin is an ether (*qi* 氣) of the ill toxins of the four seasons that is responded to by humans. Its symptoms arise at the nose, face, ears, neck, and throat, as red swelling without heads; it sometimes congeals as nodules [*jiehe* 結核] with roots. It causes people to abhor cold [*zeng han* 憎寒], to be feverish, their head to hurt and their limbs to hurt. In severe cases they are confused and disturbed, and their throats are blocked. People who do not recognize it take it to be Cold-Damage [disorder], and immediately take antidotes. In a day or two the swelling-ether increases; only then do they realize, and call a doctor of sores to examine it. Now, anciently there were no prescriptions for or discourses on this disease. The world vulgarly assimilates it to Cinnabar Tumour; the family of the sick person hates to call it Seasonal Toxin, bitterly afraid of the contagion [that this would imply]. [But] if one checks the medical classics [for Cinnabar Tumour], they talk of the body suddenly passing through a transformation [and turning] red, looking as if painted with cinnabar: it is this that is called Cinnabar Toxin; it is produced by the ill toxin of wind heat and is [also] called Cinnabar Tumour. It is very different from Seasonal Toxin. For Seasonal Toxin responds to an irregular ether (*buzheng zhi qi* 不正之氣) of the four seasons. When it first emerges, its appearance is like Cold Damage; but within five to seven days it can kill a person. To treat it one must distinguish it precisely. [...He goes on to discuss its diagnosis by pulse and various prescriptions to treat it.][64]

Here again "nodules with roots"—of a kind specifically likely to make the patient's family call on a doctor specializing in sores—appear incorporated into the older symptomatology (as above, Luo Tianyi on the 1202 epidemic) of generalized face/head swelling ("swelling without heads") and throat closure. In this instance a sequence seems to be suggested: fever, chills (abhorrence of cold), and head and muscle aches come first, while the passage "in a day or two the swelling-ether increases, and only then do they[...]call a doctor of sores" suggests that the sores ("nodules with roots"), as a manifestation of the increase in swelling-ether, follow the other symptoms. This sequence—more generalized bodily symptoms preceding buboes—is in fact quite characteristic of bubonic plague. It also seems significant that throat closure here is said to occur only in some patients ("in severe cases"), thus disaggregating a complex of symptoms that one might otherwise read as universally appearing together. Elsewhere, Qi prescribes a

---

63 Luo Tianyi, *Weisheng baojian*, 9:373–74. (Not cited by Fan or by Cao and Li.)

64 Qi Dezhi, *Waike jingyi*, j. *shang*: 84–86.

single decoction designed to treat both Seasonal Toxin and Big Head, again recognizably describing them as producing sores: "In recent times, those suffering from this disease have transmitted it by contagion, often leading to premature death. [...]On the whole, it is quite similar to Cold Damage; among [its cases] are some that may be lanced or cut to produce blood; there are also some that after a time spoil and erode producing pus."[65] Note that Qi composed both these passages without ever using the still-novel term *geda*.

In the years before or after Qi wrote, as we have seen, a Yuan-period physician (possibly a Buddhist monk) known to us simply as Shiyuan (or possibly Shi Yuan)[66] (item 15) had reproduced Mr. Yang's description of the 1138–1149 epidemics (item 4); but he added a disease name and a symptom name that Mr. Yang's own words had never mentioned: "Seasonal-Epidemic Swelling-Toxin Illness of Lumps/Sores" (*shiyi geda zhongdu bing* 時疫疙瘩腫毒病), and he placed this under the more general heading "Seasonal-Epidemic Lumps/Sores" (*shiyi geda* 時疫疙瘩). The correspondence to Luo Tianyi's use of the terms "seasonal epidemic" and "swelling toxin" in his discussion of "A Prescription for Lumps/Sores of Seasonal Toxin" is close, though Shiyuan chooses a disease name that combines the same elements in a different way. The complete item is as follows:

> *Seasonal-Epidemic Lumps/Sores* (*geda*). This "Seasonal-Epidemic Toxin-Swelling Illness of Lumps/Sores" is something of which there is no mention in the discussions in ancient prescription books. The men of antiquity did not have this illness; thus their prescriptions did not mention it. Only in the Zhenglong period [1156–1161] in Mr. Yang's *Prescriptions for Rescue and Aid* [*Zhengji fang*] does it say: "Between the Tianjuan [1138–1140] and Huangtong [1141–1149] periods, first north of the ridges, next in Taiyuan, finally in Yan(zhou) and Ji(zhou), the mountain villages and quarters suffered severely from this affliction, which down to today has not ended. It is transmitted from one [person] to another, in many cases leading to death; there are even some who [when faced with it] do not protect their families. In presentation it is similar to Thunder Head, swelling the throat and neck. If it attacks internally, the throat is blocked, and water and medicine pass with difficulty. If it attacks externally, the head and face are like [those of] an ox, the eye and ear orifices fill up, and looking and listening are both negated, shutting off hearing and seeing. When the illness is serious it endangers life."[67] [What follows are treatment recommendations, whether Mr. Yang's own or Shiyuan's is unclear.]

---

65 Qi Dezhi, *Waike, xia* 下:31.

66 In fact, it is uncertain whether in fact we should read "Shiyuan" in the title *Shiyuan duanxiao fang* 施圓端效方 as a personal name and thus translate it *Shiyuan's Proper and Effective Prescriptions*, as I have done here. In principle, Shi 施 could be a surname and Yuan 圓 a given name, though it would be unusual for a surname / given name combination to appear within a book title. Alternatively, *shiyuan* could plausibly be a Buddhist compound, combining *shi* "to make donations, to be charitable" and *yuan* "complete, perfect, completion, perfection," thus "to be perfectly charitable," in which case the combination becomes plausible as a monk's name. But on that reading, *Proper and Effective Prescriptions for Perfect Charity* would become a plausible title as well, since knowledge of medical prescriptions on a gentleman's part was often seen as a facet of his charitable function toward a wider social world.

67 The entire passage from Shiyuan's work survives only through its inclusion, along with thousands of other excerpts from previous medical texts both surviving and lost, in the 1447 Korean compilation *Categorized Collection of Medical Prescriptions* (*Uibang yuch'wi* 醫方類) (item

The passage beginning "Between the Tianjuan[...]," of course, is quoted from the ca. 1156 account of Mr. Yang, which I have already given above (p. 17); here it is worth seeing it in its Yuan, as opposed to Jin, context. As my note indicates, it is unclear where we should see Mr. Yang's discussion as ending and Shiyuan's as resuming (if anywhere); I end where I do because a full and rounded disease description seems to end there. Even whether Shiyuan is quoting or merely paraphrasing Mr. Yang is uncertain.

What is clear is that nothing that can be taken as Mr. Yang's own words makes any mention of lumps or sores, and this goes for the continuation that discusses treatment as well (not quoted here). Rather, Shiyuan seems to be making the same move as the predecessors we have already seen (Wang Haogu, Luo Tianyi, Qi Dezhi if he writes before Shiyuan) by incorporating lumps or sores (*geda*, in all these authors except Qi) into an older disease description that had not previously included them—and for the sake of the historical sequence I am trying to reconstruct here, it is crucial to see that it had not—but rather had emphasized throat closure and head swelling. Looking for historical precedent for a disease he is immediately concerned with and finding none in "ancient" works, Shiyuan reaches back for a Jin precedent in the epidemics Mr. Yang had described a century or more before. We do not know that any earlier author such as Wang or Luo, or possibly later author such as Qi, was aware of Mr. Yang's work or saw it in the same light; but each of them similarly incorporated a newly-encountered symptom into one or another previously-described epidemic disease. The same can be said of the Ming-dynasty medical author Zhu Su (item 18), whose *Prescriptions for General Aid* (*Puji fang* 普濟方) incorporates Shiyuan's entire discussion, and thus the full name "Seasonal-Epidemic Toxin-Swelling Illness of Lumps/Sores", including the material from Mr. Yang, under the simpler disease name "Swelling Toxin" (*zhongdu* 腫毒); but interestingly, his own introductory discussion mentions fever and chills but not throat closure.[68]

Epidemic Categories after the Mongols' Arrival: Summing Up

In examining this series of Jin, Yuan, and Ming discussions, two points deserve focus. The first is the recurrent suggestion—arguably already implied by the unsettled and shifting terminology of disease names—that the diseases under discussion are new, or that they present deceptively as some other and older category of illness. Zhang Congzheng, if in fact he belongs in this list, assimilates what he has seen or heard of to "a miasmic pestilence," and objects to his contemporaries' taking it as a manifestation of cold—suggesting that they are seeing it as Cold Damage Disorder. Li Gao, as we have seen, tells us that the doctors present at the 1232 epidemic in Kaifeng were mistaking the disease for Cold Damage.[69] In fact, he sees existing medical theories as incapable of explaining the disease in question and devises a new system, "Internal Damage," to cope with it. Qi Dezhi writes of Seasonal Toxin that "anciently there were no prescriptions for or discourses on this disease," that "people who do not recognize it take it for

---

19), reprinted in China in 1981 under the exactly equivalent Chinese title *Yifang leiju*, here 179:419.

68 Zhu Su, *Puji fang*, 279:1a–21a.

69 Li Gao, *Nei wai shang bian huo lun*, 8.

Cold Damage," that "the world customarily assimilates [the sores] to Cinnabar Tumour," and furthermore that patients' families are frightened of a diagnosis as Seasonal Toxin because of the contagion it implies. Shiyuan tells us that Seasonal-Epidemic Lumps/ Sores "is something of which there is no mention in the discussions in ancient prescription books" because "the men of antiquity did not have this illness." Again and again, that is, we see explicit declarations or implicit indications that a disease is previously unknown or else misrecognized and thus likely to be wrongly shoehorned by other physicians into existing categories.

My argument is that the incorporation of *geda* and other terms for lumps or sores into disease categories where they had never been noted before, such as Big Head, Thunder Head, Seasonal Toxin, and Seasonal Epidemic, is methodologically and logically closely akin to such shoehorning, even when physicians see similar procedures in others' work as mistakes. In fact, they are testifying to the tendency of middle-period Chinese physicians to do what I am arguing they themselves are doing.

But if (in our terms) plague was what they were dealing with, why would medical authors carry forward, from earlier diseases like Big Head, symptoms that would not seem characteristic of plague, such as throat-closure or general and dramatic swelling of the head and neck, and simply add purulent sores to them? Perhaps partly because epidemicity, high fever, and frequent and rapid fatality seemed to them the primary characteristics of either disease, and the ones most suggestive of the underlying processes that ultimately should determine treatment under urgent circumstances; perhaps because, to their minds, large swellings on the neck (and elsewhere), a typical site for buboes, were easily assimilated to general swelling of the neck (and head), especially causally in terms of "swelling-toxin" and the like; but also partly because, as I have already suggested, they assumed that disease entities were mutable, responsive to the vagaries of environment and of individual constitution, and that since a symptomatic description of a disease could never be either exhaustive or exclusive, one should not expect to find every symptom of a previously-described disease in each future occurrence of it. Perhaps a disease description that we would read as implying "look for epidemicity, high fever, rapid fatality, generalized swelling of the head and neck, and purulent lumps" would instead imply, to them, "look for epidemicity, high fever, rapid fatality, generalized swelling of the head and neck, *and/or* purulent lumps." What might make all this especially likely is that buboes emerge rather late in the course of a plague case, so that for several days a doctor would have only more generalized symptoms to base an initial diagnosis on. (Qi Dezhi's account suggests this.) Further, in those early stages of plague, according to authorities of our own time, sometimes "the face appears red, swollen, and masklike"—never producing the dramatic "head like an ox" described for Big Head, but perhaps capable of being taken by a doctor as an early step toward it.[70]

In sum, I suggest that doctors of the Yuan, the special case of Li Gao aside, reacted to an encounter with plague by thinking they were dealing with that particular year's, or that particular cosmological phase's, symptomatologically new and interesting version of Big Head / Thunder Head / Seasonal Epidemic / Cold Damage—and found this

---

70 Nikoforov et al., "Plague" (2016), 295.

a natural and unproblematic way to think about disease. The new symptom certainly registered, was catalogued, and could call for special treatments of its own; but it did not, except to Li Gao, demand a new disease category when several older categories of febrile and often-fatal epidemic were available.

A second point is that the term *geda* 疙瘩, which we have seen repeatedly here, and which I have been translating noncommittally as simply "lumps/sores," is an entirely new term in surviving Chinese epidemic discourse, and barely known in other Chinese medical discourse, either. As applied to epidemics, we have seen it twice in Wang Haogu, in (perhaps) 1253 and 1264; in Xu Guozhen in 1267; three times in Luo Tianyi as of 1281; in Shiyuan ca. 1300; and three times in Zhu Su in 1406, both reproducing Shiyuan and independently. It is very striking, and surely significant, that two of the authors most responsible for the introduction of *geda* into epidemic discourse in the sources traced here, Wang Haogu and Luo Tianyi, had been students of Li Gao and would presumably have had the opportunity to hear from him about the 1232 Kaifeng epidemic in more detail than we can hear from him now. All this is reason to examine the history of *geda* more closely.

The Sudden Rise of the *Geda*

Until the Yuan, the word *geda* hardly exists in surviving writings. Before the Jin- and Yuan-period works I have been discussing so far, *geda* 疙瘩[71] or its synonym *gedan* 疙疸 (also pronounceable *geda*)[72] had occurred with a medical meaning just three times in the surviving Chinese written record, in two medical works of the Tang and Song dynasties.[73] (With a non-medical meaning it had occurred just another five times.)[74] The term

---

71 疙瘩 is not the only pair of characters that is used to convey the term in this pronunciation: the *Hanyu da cidian* lists several alternatives, and the most prominent pairings that appear in the digital databases I have consulted are those in which either the silk radical (thus 纥縺, changing the phonetic element of the second character as well) or the flesh radical (making the first character 肐) replaces the illness radical in both characters. The second character of the flesh-radical version is unavailable in my Chinese font, but 月 + 荅 will convey it.

72 The *Hanyu da cidian* treats the words as synonyms, and in my searches of the *Wenyuange Siku quanshu dianziban* and *Zhongguo jiben gujiku* 中國基本古籍庫 digital databases they have appeared interchangeable.

73 Sun Simiao, *Yinhai jingwei*, 1:13a and 2:10a. (*Zhongguo jiben gujiku* citations 1:10 and 2:27.) Chen Yan, *Sanyin jiyi bingzheng fang lun*, 15:2b–3a.

74 In modern usage, the word can carry a large number of non-medical meanings (according to the *Hanyu da cidian*), ranging from "knot" through "round or ball-shaped object" through "lump, piece" to "mound, knoll" and even, in regional speech, simply "point in place or time;" but also to "trouble, disagreement, doubtful point." It can also refer to a lump-shaped pasta fried or used in a soup, in English often called a "dumpling knot." (See the excellent recipe for dumpling knots [*mian geda* 麵疙瘩, literally "pasta *geda*"] provided by Ellen Schrecker [with John Schrecker] in her *Mrs. Chiang's Szechwan Cookbook: Szechwan Home Cooking* [New York: Harper and Row, 1976; reissued 1987], 302–6.) More or less this full range would be easy to understand etymologically if "knot" was the original referent, tending in one direction toward "lump" and related notions and in a different direction toward "doubtful point" (as in English "knotty"), "disagreement," "trouble," then more or less explodes in the medical discourse of Yuan, Ming, and Qing, increasing steadily in frequency from one dynasty to the next. The character of Yuan usage is unique, however: about half of all medical mentions of *geda* in Yuan times record it as a symptom of *epidemic* disease. This will shrink to less than a fifth in the Ming and will rise significantly again, though only to nearly a third, in the period between the Qing conquest and 1800. This suggests that the explosion of the term in general was itself a response to encounters with purulent lumps in the epidemics of the Jin–Yuan: that, as doctors acquired the habit of calling a certain sort of thing a *geda* when they observed it in epidemics, the name was then transferred logically to comparable symptoms in non-epidemic diseases;[75] and that this application became more and more common as the particular sort of epidemic disease observed in Jin and Yuan retreated in subsequent decades and centuries—though perhaps not without recurrence.

Charts 2.1–5 illustrate the historical rise and flourishing of the medical *geda*. Chart 2.1 maps the occurrences of the word over the Tang, Song, Yuan, Ming, and Qing dynasties. (It begins with Tang because the word does not occur in surviving sources before then.) To normalize for the different lengths of dynasties, the chart measures the occurrences per fifty-year period. (I should note that the Song bar, which shrinks to a bare line [or less] at this scale, represents one occurrence, not zero.) In Chart 2.1 overleaf, we see the rise of the medical *geda*, almost out of nowhere, and its continuous growth in frequency into modern times. Chart 2.2 shows that the arc of its application to epidemics specifically is different: here the Yuan and Qing come to the fore, and the Ming fades somewhat into the background. Chart 2.3 shows this even more clearly by mapping the *proportion* of all *geda* mentions that refer to epidemics: in this case, the Yuan absolutely stands out, though the Qing still shows a significantly higher proportion than the Ming.

These charts support the inference that it was the initial encounter with epidemics manifesting purulent lumps that stimulated the new explosion of the term in medical discourse; but that already in the Yuan, to some degree, and more and more in the Ming

---

and so on. (The etymology gains some appeal from its similarity to that of "node" from Latin *nodus*, a knot.) This, however, must remain speculative for now, since in the earliest textual records of the term, in Tang and Song, the only uses that appear are (in chronological order) the medical sense, of a lump on or under the skin; a sense as some form of food served in restaurants; and an obscure usage having to do with some part of the body of crickets and other insects (possibly a bump or knob on the head or on the end of the antennae). For the culinary usage, very possibly referring to the same sort of lump-like pasta as today, then being served in restaurants in the Song capital, see Meng Yuanlao 孟元老 (fl. ca. 1136), *Dongjing menghua lu*, 4:6a, in the article entitled "restaurants" (*shidian* 食店). For the entomological usage, see Jia Sidao (1213–1275), *Cuzhi jing*, *shang* 上:7 (*Zhongguo jiben gujiku* citation *shang* 上: 16a), in the article entitled *Lun ding* 論頂; and his *Qiuqiong pu, xia* 下:3a, 8a, and 9b (*Zhongguo jiben gujiku* citation *xia*: 6; 8, line 2; and 8, line 33), in the articles respectively titled *Xiang sheng shangdeng* 項生上等, *Zhenhuang zeng shi* 真黃增釋, and *Zhenzi zeng shi* 真紫增釋. Note that, given the author's dates, the Jia Sidao passages are probably later than the earliest Jin–Yuan passages discussed so far.

75 The word "bubo" itself in modern biomedical discourse is also not unique to plague, but occurs in relation to tuberculosis and to syphilis, and can be applied to an isolated symptom as well: essentially any purulent swelling of a lymph node is a bubo. I am suggesting that the same extension of referent happened over time with medical usages of *geda*.

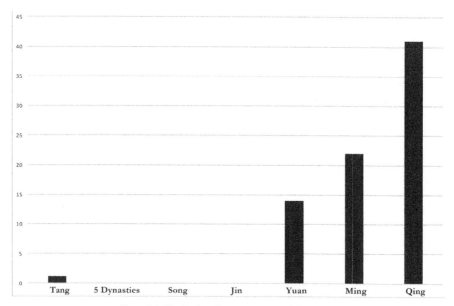

Chart 2.1. Medical *geda* mentions per fifty years,
by dynasty (Tang to 1800).

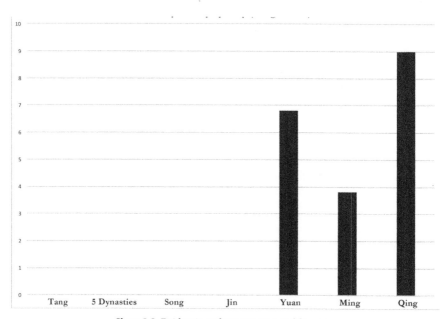

Chart 2.2. Epidemic *geda* mentions per fifty years,
by dynasty (Tang to 1800).

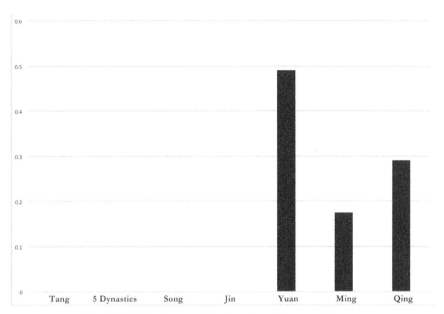

Chart 2.3. Epidemic proportion of *geda* mentions per fifty years,
by dynasty (Tang to 1800).

and Qing, the term expanded its application to include non-epidemic phenomena. The charts might also suggest that while epidemic *geda* never faded from view (or perhaps from memory), they grew significantly less salient for medical authors in the Ming and then significantly regained salience in the Qing. Does this signal a recurrence of *geda*-bearing epidemics in the Qing or at the Ming–Qing transition? Further on, I will offer another way of looking at these data that may hint in that direction.

It is important, however, to get one possible alternative interpretation of the data out of the way. Might the number of occurrences of the term *geda*, even when normalized for length of dynasty, simply or largely reflect the distribution of sources across the dynasties? Surviving Chinese historical sources generally increase dynasty by dynasty: is this all we are seeing in the Yuan–Ming–Qing picture? Charts 2.4 and 2.5 address this by comparing the temporal distribution of *geda* with that of another, much more common and much older medical term for a sore, *chuang*; and for this purpose, it is appropriate to extend the question all the way back to the Han dynasty. Note that because *chuang* is a much commoner term, the charts' scales are different. (Note also that I omit Ming and Qing from these two charts because the numbers for *chuang* become so high that one cannot easily display all the dynasties on a single scale.)

Readers familiar with the sources for premodern Chinese history will see that the distribution of references to *chuang* from the early imperial through middle imperial dynasties reflects the sheer availability of sources much more closely than the distribution of *geda* does. The enormous increase in Five Dynasties–Song sources of course

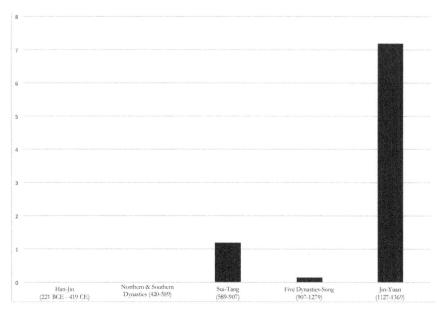

Chart 2.4. Medical *geda* mentions per fifty years,
by dynasty (Han through Yuan).

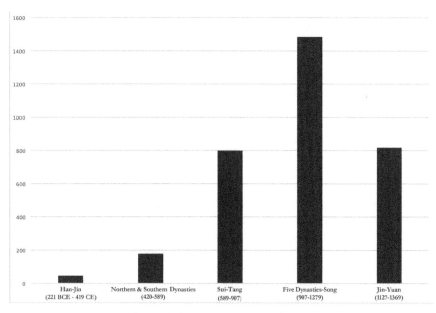

Chart 2.5. *Chuang* mentions per fifty years,
by dynasty (Han through Yuan).

reflects the relatively sudden rise of printed books in the period; the falloff in Jin–Yuan is in line with our broader awareness that the printed source base for almost half of China, the north, shrinks dramatically with the fall of Northern Song and still more with the fall of Jin. For *geda*, the almost complete silence in the Song and explosive increase in the Yuan stand in the sharpest possible contrast to the *chuang* picture, as well as to the relative quantities of books from the periods. Setting the pictures side by side here makes it crystal clear that something new really did happen in the Yuan: after being a marginal term in any of its applications before the 1250s, *geda* very suddenly drew the interest of medical authors. The previous charts have already shown that, in Yuan, a uniquely high proportion of that new interest was directed toward epidemics.

What Was a *Geda*?

But what, in this period and these usages, was a *geda*? In modern usage, even as a medical term, *geda* can refer to any subcutaneous lump or sore down to the size of a pimple; and the non-medical uses evidenced in Tang, Song, and Yuan texts—ranging from a topographical feature we might call a small hill,[76] through a food item probably comparable to a small wonton,[77] down to a knot in raw strands encountered when unreeling a silkworm cocoon,[78] or an uncertain insect body part[79]—hardly serve to narrow down size. The two Tang and Song medical authors who mention *geda* both use it to refer to a stye on an eyelid, so a very small size was clearly possible at that time. As buboes are generally a good deal bigger than a stye or a pimple, one would like to know what phenomena Jin–Yuan doctors thought deserved the name *geda*. Unfortunately, medical texts mention *geda* often but describe them rarely, and descriptions are rarely complete. In particular, Yuan, Ming, and Qing sources are much more likely to specify a *geda*'s colour and its purulence than its size. What we do have, however, suggests that a Jin–Yuan *geda* was no mere pimple.

The most complete description appears in a source hard to date precisely: it is most likely of Yuan date but could conceivably belong to late Southern Song. Surprisingly, the source is a book not on human medicine but on horse-doctoring, the *Pasture-Director's Collection for Contented Steeds* (*Simu anji ji* 司牧安驥集). Possibly of Tang origin and known to have been promulgated in a four-chapter revised edition in 1135, under the Jin's Shandong puppet state of Qi, the book had acquired a fifth chapter by 1192. By Yuan times, it existed in an eight-chapter version, with three new chapters appended to the 1192 redaction. The passages relevant here appear in the sixth chapter of that eight-chapter edition, so we are dealing with material that dates either to the Yuan or to the post-1192 years of the Southern Song: in either case, not terribly far from the middle decades of the thirteenth century when *geda* began to be linked to epi-

---

76 Zhou Boqi, *Hucong ji*, 26a.

77 Meng Yuanlao, j. 4.

78 [Sinongsi], *Nongsang jiyao*, 4:26a and 27b–28b.

79 Jia Sidao, *Cuzhi jing* and *Qiuqiong pu*, as cited in note 74.

demic disease.[80] In the *Collection* we see what a late Song or Yuan horse doctor thought deserved to be called a *geda*. The term appears in two verses of mnemonic doggerel in a series of such verses dealing with the origins of different sorts of horse-ailments. My own doggerel conveys, I hope, both their basic content and their tone.

> The puffy-swollen *geda*'s as big as a polo ball.
> As swelling-*qi* pervades the body, sweat of course will fall.
> Puffy swelling, basically, we get from rising heat;
> The doctor must remember this within his heart's seat.
> The *geda*'s upper surface with needle fine he'll pop;
> From sore's mouth at once then the fatty oil will slop.[81]
> Next the cooling drug of slender evodia pour:
> In a moment end the sickness that was there before.

> 虛腫胲[月+荅]大如毬
> 腫氣通身汗自流
> 虛腫元来熱上得
> 醫人湏記在心頭
> 胲[月+荅]上面碎針破
> 瘡口立便潤脂油
> 更用消黃凉藥嗶
> 從来有病便湏休

> The sweat comes out and soaks the trunk; the *geda* polo ball
> Comes to a head which, rubbed and popped, may fatty oil recall.
> Rub and pop: the fatty oil will stink like rotting meat;
> The doctor must remember this within his heart's seat.
> Know this illness: if you wait to minister and cure,
> If death is not in summertime, then early fall for sure.
> The truth within the former Classics now you will regard:
> Confronting this, when fate's used up, to herd the dead is hard.

> 汗出渾身胲[月+荅]毬
> 發米擦破似脂油
> 擦破脂油腥爛臭

---

80 For the bibliographic history of the *Collection*, the foreword to the 2001 annotated edition published by the Chinese Agricultural Publishing House is very useful, and I follow their judgment that the sixth chapter is "at latest" of Yuan date. See Deng and He, eds., *Simu anji ji* (2001), 1–5 for the former and 311 for the latter. For the text of the poems in this version, see 321 and 340, songs 22 and 64.

81 The *Collection*'s modern editors argue that "fatty oil" (*zhiyou* 脂油) here refers to the salve the doctor applies to the sore after lancing it, and would thus translate *run* 潤, which I render as "slop," as "imbibe" or "absorb" instead: something like "The sore's mouth will then at once absorb the fatty oil." See Deng and He, eds., *Simu anji ji*, 321n2. However, the second poem makes it clear that the substance in question merely *looks like* "fatty oil": I've rendered that line as "may fatty oil recall" for the sake of the rhyme, but a literal translation would be simply "resembles fatty oil" (*si zhi you* 似脂油). To my mind, the allusion is clearly to a pus-like exudate; where the second poem handles this with straightforward simile, the first resorts to metaphor. The line-final rhyme throughout both poems is -*u* (or -*ou* in modern pronunciation depending on the phonological context), and it seems clear the author has selected "fatty oil," *zhi you* 脂油, as his term for the pus largely because it will rhyme with *qiu* 球 ("polo ball") and the other line-ending words (*liu* 流, *tou* 頭, and *xiu* 休 in the first poem; and *qiu* 球 again, *chou* 臭, *tou* 頭 again, and *mu* 牧 in the second).

瞖人莫記在心頭
識其此病休治療
夏天不死在初秋
先經論裡知端的
交它命盡死難牧.[82]

Of course, I am not suggesting that the *geda* mentioned here are the same thing as buboes caused by plague; there is little evidence that horses are likely to contract plague, and in any case these sores are "all over the body," not in the mere two or three major lymphatic sites that buboes typically inhabit.[83] We have seen that other Yuan sources sometimes used the word *geda* in non-epidemic contexts, and clearly this one is doing so too. The point is rather what kind of thing one (probably) Yuan doctor thought a *geda* was, and the text makes the answer beautifully clear: a purulent swelling, rupturable by lancing or by pressure, and about the size of a polo ball (see Figure 2.1).[84] Even reduced in proportion to the size difference between a horse and a human, this is no mere pimple; and if a physician, whoever his patient, had thought the modal *geda* in humans was pimple-sized, he surely would not have borrowed the term for something this large on a horse.

Later Yuan and Ming descriptions, though rare, also report something of substantial size when describing the *geda*. Shen Zhou 沈周 (1427–1509), in his *New Reports from the Guest's Seat* (*Kezuo xinwen* 客座新聞), offers the case of a man who suffered *geda* "like purple apricots" scattered about his body.[85] In his *Categorized Cases of Famous Physicians* (*Mingyi leian* 名醫類案, prefaced 1549, Wang Guan 汪瓘 (1503–1565) reports a patient whose two *geda* on his neck were "like pigs' kidneys."[86] Pigs' kidneys are not very different in size from human kidneys: about four inches long. Such a bubo would be something extraordinary, and perhaps Wang reports its size precisely because it is unusual: but its size does not remove it from the category of *geda* for him.[87] (By con-

---

82 Deng and He, eds., *Simu anji ji*, j. 6.

83 Alexandre Yersin (discoverer of the plague bacillus), in the course of trying to develop a plague vaccine, "was able to obtain a certain degree of immunity in a horse by injecting small quantities of the plague bacillus subcutaneously, and afterwards, as this produced suppuration, by making intravenous injections of the plague bacillus, these injections being repeated from time to time as the temperature went down, the glandular enlargements and joint tenderness disappeared, and the animal came to its normal condition." That is, Yersin produced suppuration, fever, and glandular enlargements, all standard features of human plague, in a horse (anonymous 1897 article in the *British Medical Journal* entitled "The Plague. The Antitoxin Serum"). Thus, horses do not appear to have any preexisting plague immunity as such. In nature, however, it appears to be rare for fleas to infect horses—there is no horse-specific flea species—which probably makes their contracting plague unlikely. For Yersin's own report on this work see Yersin, "Sur la peste bubonique (sero-thérapie)."

84 From paintings of the Chinese middle period, it would appear that their polo ball was much the size of a polo ball of our time: see Fong, "Tang Tomb Murals," Figure 9b.

85 Shen Zhou, *Kezuo xinwen*, 10:12a (*Zhongguo jiben gujiku* citation 10:70.)

86 Wang Guan, *Mingyi leian*, 6:7a.

87 One might speculate that "like pig's kidneys" was only supposed to convey shape, not size; but if they were pimple-sized but roughly kidney-shaped, it would be more natural for Wang Kentang to describe them as "like beans."

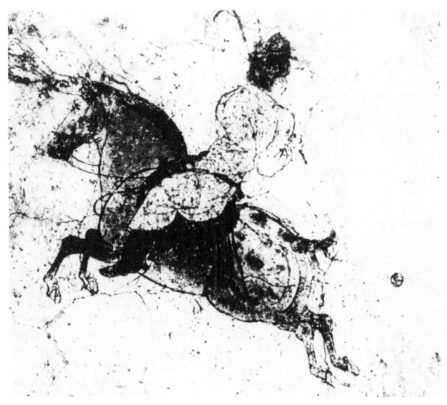

Figure 2.1. Polo player with a ball the size of a horse's *geda*.
Detail from a mural on the west wall of the path to the tomb of Prince Zhanghuai
(Li Xian 李賢, 655–684) in Chang'an (now Xian), CE 706. After *Tang Li Xian mu bi hua*
唐李賢墓壁畫, compiled by the Shaanxi Provincial Museum (Shaanxi sheng bowuguan
陝西省博物館) and the Shaanxi Cultural Relics Conservation Committee (Shaanxi sheng wenwu
guanli weiyuanhui 陝西省文物管理委员会) (Beijing: Wenwu chubanshe, 1974), plate 16.

trast, imagine the unlikelihood of calling a four-inch lump on a human face a "pimple.")
In his *Complete Writings of Jingyue* (*Jingyue quanshu* 景岳全書), Zhang Jiebin 張介賓
(1563–1640) describes a man with a *geda* "the size of a coin."[88] (Bear in mind that premodern Chinese coins were roughly an inch and a quarter, or 3 cm, across.) The late-
Ming author Chen Shigong 陳實功 (fl. 1615–1617), in one of a series of songs on *yin*-
pattern illness in his *Direct Lineage of Internal Medicine* (*Waike zhengzong* 外科正宗),
describes the process of a *geda*'s emergence, in which it is initially like a grain of millet: "When it first arises, on the *jihai* day of the tenth month, he doesn't know it is a
sore / With the form of a grain of millet, the *geda* is dormant (僵)." But he goes on to

---

88 Zhang Jiebin, *Jingyue quanshu*, 25:21b.

tell us that, seven days later, "the sore's root is flat and big."[89] The *Humane and Upright Record* (*Renduan lu* 仁端錄), a 1644 collection by Xu Qian 徐謙 and Chen Gui 陳葵, also mentions *geda* the size of a millet grain but treats them as just one in a range of types. Yu Chang 喻昌 (1585–1664), a pioneer of the new theoretical tendency of early Qing that emphasized "warm disease" (*wenbing* 溫病), touches on "*Geda* epidemic" (*geda wen* 疙瘩瘟) in his *Essays on Communing with the Past* (*Shanglun pian* 尚論篇) of 1648, describing it as an illness "with redness and swelling all over the body that produces lumps like tumours [*liu* 瘤]"[90]—again suggesting something of at least middling size.

It is not till the eighteenth century that one begins to find descriptions of pimple-sized *geda*. Wu Qian 吳謙, in his 1742 compilation *A Metal Mirror for the Medical Lineage* (*Yizong quanlan* 醫宗金鑒), reproduces Chen Shigong's song, with its millet-sized *geda* as only an early dormant stage;[91] but elsewhere, in several places, he describes *geda* straightforwardly as grain-sized,[92] and in another place says that they are the size of a grain of rice (if small) or the size of a bean (if large).[93] Yet he also writes of *geda* that are "like a peach, or like a duck or goose egg."[94] It may be that, in the later years of the late-imperial era, the scope of the term *geda* once again expanded to include lumps as small as the styes it had first labelled in the Tang, and perhaps this culminated in the modern use of *geda* for "pimple." However, Wu Qian's evidence shows that it had not yet lost its application to much larger lesions in 1742.

The sources testify much more often to two other characteristics of *geda*, colour and purulence, than they do to size. Again and again we are told that, if lanced or if ruptured naturally, a *geda* exudes pus; occasionally, the description adds or substitutes blood or clear fluid (perhaps lymph).[95] As to colour, most sources mention purple, some purple-black, some red.[96] In fact, it is only in mentioning colour that the descriptions in Ming and Qing texts enlarge upon what the author of the *Pasture-Director's Collection for Contented Steeds* had already described in the Yuan. From Yuan through Qing, a *geda* was or could be a large or middle-sized lump, whose colour reflected inflammation, and which often yielded pus when ruptured. Every part of this description would have made *geda* an apt name for a plague bubo as attested in fourteenth-century Europe and observable up to the present day.

---

89 Chen Shigong, *Waike zhengzong*, 1:52 (*Zhongguo jiben gujiku* citation 1:12.)

90 Yu Chang, *Shanglun pian*, *shou* 首:32a. According to Wiseman and Feng, *Practical Dictionary of Chinese Medicine* (1998–2012), a *liu* 瘤—what I translate as "tumour" above—is "a sudden swelling in the skin and flesh that is as large as a plum at onset." If Yu Chang was using the term in the same way, he was talking about something not unlike a bubo.

91 Wu Qian, *Yizong quanlan*, 61:43b–44a (*Zhongguo jiben gujiku* citation 61:1027.).

92 Wu Qian, *Yizong quanlan*, 61:52a, 69:18b, 74:22b. (*Zhongguo jiben gujiku* citations 61:1031, 69:1190, 74:1265 respectively.) (The last makes the *geda* the size of the seed of a string bean.)

93 Wu Qian, *Yizong quanlan*, 63:66a. (*Zhongguo jiben gujiku* citation 63:1087.)

94 Wu Qian, *Yizong quanlan*, 6810a. (*Zhongguo jiben gujiku* citation 68:1173.)

95 Citations could be legion, and there is not room for them all here: probably something more than half the medical mentions of *geda* in Yuan, Ming, and Qing sources in the *Wenyuange Siku quanshu dianziban* or *Zhongguo jiben gujiku* digital databases explicitly mention purulence.

96 Again, citations would exceed my space.

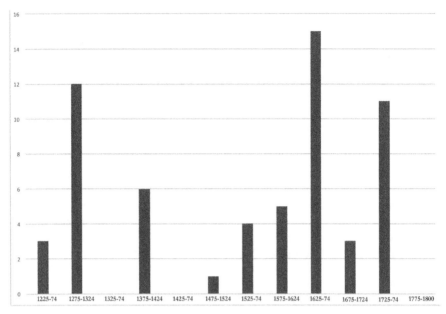

Chart 2.6. Epidemic *geda* mentions,
by fifty-year period (Yuan to 1800).

Here we may return to the temporal distribution of the *geda* associated with epidemics in the Ming and Qing. Chart 2.6 divides the nearly six hundred years from around the fall of the Jin to 1800 into fifty-year periods and charts the mentions of epidemic *geda* per period.[97] This is a much finer way to divide the data than by dynasty, and it shows something quite striking: a peak at the Ming–Qing divide—the fifty years from 1625 through 1674—that is even higher than the Yuan peak of 1275–1324.

Of course, the Qing is much richer in sources than the Yuan, while the early Ming—included in the 1325–1374 and 1375–1424 periods here—is much less so than either. If one were to adjust these period numbers in proportion to the numbers of surviving sources for each period, the Ming–Qing peak would undoubtedly drop below the Yuan peak again; but the fact that the 1625–1674 peak is the highest in post-Yuan Chinese history jibes very nicely with a view current in the field (though by no means uncontroversial) that at least some of the epidemics of the late Ming and Ming–Qing transition

---

97 It is important to remember that the records examined throughout this article, and thus charted here, are with a very few exceptions *not* records of specific dated epidemic outbreaks, but rather the mentions of *geda* as a symptom associated with *categories* of epidemic disease, in medical compilations that often make no reference to specific dated events at all. The dates here are dates of publication or authorship of works mentioning *geda*. One might thus expect a certain time lag between the occurrence of a symptom in an actual epidemic and its registration, in the abstract, as an epidemic symptom in medical compilations.

may have been plague. Cao Shuji proposed this in 1997,[98] and both Marta Hanson[99] and Timothy Brook[100] have recently found it plausible. And of course, the seventeenth century also saw the largest-scale recurrence of plague in Europe: the second hump, as it were, of the Second Plague Pandemic. Here, the new Qing category of *geda wen*, "*geda* epidemic," becomes salient. We have seen Yu Chang discussing this in 1648, but it had previously appeared in 1642, in the work of the founder of "warm disease" theory, Wu Youxing 吳有性. This is all the more intriguing since, in rethinking the epidemic disease categories and theory of his time, Wu (as Marta Hanson has shown) saw himself as responding to the late Ming epidemics—very much as Li Gao had devised "Internal Damage" theory in response to the Kaifeng epidemic of 1232 and the North China epidemics of the preceding two decades.[101]

Caution is needed here. The data mapped in Chart 2.6 above are complicated by the tendency of medical authors and compilers to copy or echo the work of previous authorities: appearance of an epidemic symptom in a medical work need not *necessarily* mean that the author had seen it or that a relevant epidemic had occurred recently.[102] Some of the lesser peaks in the chart may simply reflect periodic bouts of reorganization or republication of older material; and that may feed higher peaks, too (apart from the initial Yuan peak). There is also the complication that while Yu Chang, as we have seen, had described "*geda* epidemic" as characterized by tumour-like lumps on the body, Wu Youxing described it rather differently as involving "goiter and intermittent fever" (*yingjie* 瘿疥).[103] Now *ying* 瘿, conventionally translated as "goiter," involves large swellings on the neck, and perhaps a doctor could see buboes and classify them in these terms; but intermittent fever sounds quite unlike plague. Of course we need not assume that Wu Youxing, who was undertaking a conceptual and theoretical reorganization of epidemic disease, had actually seen all of

---

98 See again Cao, "Shuyi liuxing" (1997). In her earlier study of epidemics at the Ming–Qing transition, Helen Dunstan, while appropriately cautious and skeptical, was willing to entertain the possibility that those in North China in 1643–1644 were plague: see Dunstan, "The Late Ming Epidemics" (1973), 19–23. Carol Benedict was more thoroughly skeptical in her *Bubonic Plague in Nineteenth-Century China* (1996), 10–11. Long before Cao Shuji wrote, Wu Lien-teh, a founding figure of both plague treatment and plague studies in China, had included the 1640s epidemics in bis brief timeline of the "History of Plague in China," and even specifically noted Wu Youxing's (under the latter's courtesy-name Wu Youke 吳又可) category "*geda* epidemic" (*geda wen*), which he called "bubo epidemic" (Wu Lien-teh, *Plague* (1936), 11; see also 14.)

99 Hanson was kind enough to share with me a draft chapter, "The Late-Ming Epidemics," not ultimately included in her dissertation or book, in which she found Cao's claim of plague plausible for the late Ming epidemics that took place on the North China plain.

100 Brook, *The Great State* (2020), 243–44. In his earlier *The Troubled Empire* (2010), he had been skeptical of plague in the fourteenth century (65–67) but somewhat less so in the seventeenth (251); see also his "Comparative Pandemics" (2020).

101 Hanson, *Speaking of Epidemics*, 91–103.

102 Nahyan Fancy notes a similar phenomenon to the one I am suggesting: that while detailed descriptions of plague continue to appear in Arabic medical writings long past the Justinianic Plague's impact in western Asia, "their derivative writing suggests that physicians from Egypt, Syria, Iraq, and Iran did not have much direct experience with the disease": "Knowing the Signs" (2022), 36.

103 Wu Youxing, *Wenyi lun, xia* 下:2a.

the diseases he recategorized as "warm disease," or was even primarily concerned with getting individual diseases just right. Why Wu Youxing and Yu Chang, despite the latter's clear copying of the former, should describe "*geda* epidemic" so differently is still a potentially fruitful question in its own right. The question of how "*geda* epidemic," a compound term that does not appear before the seventeenth century, relates to the mentions of *geda* in association with epidemics in Yuan, and thus the question of the significance of the 1625–1674 peak, remains an intriguing question for future research.

What Did Li Gao See?

My argument so far is that the emergence of the term *geda* (and in some cases other terms for purulent sores or lumps) in Chinese medical discourse on epidemics in the thirteenth and fourteenth centuries reflects an encounter with bubonic plague: that at least some of the specific, dated epidemics that nonmedical and (less often) medical sources record were plague, and that older categories and symptom-descriptions of febrile epidemic absorbed a new disease phenomenon by adding this newly salient symptom.

But I began these pages with one apparent exception to this pattern of symptom-addition: the example of Li Gao, whose experience with the Kaifeng epidemic of 1232 motivated him (as he said in 1247) to develop an entirely new theory of epidemic disease, the "Internal Damage" (*neishang* 內傷) theory. In the continuation of the passage with which we began, Li seems to make sense of this intellectual move as a response, not to particular symptoms, but to the utter failure of conventional treatment: a response, that is, to massive and uncontrollable death. Perhaps it is the overwhelming salience of mass death itself that inclines him to give his reader next to no explicit symptomatic description of the epidemic he witnessed.

> Could all these million people have contracted wind-cold external damage [referring to Cold Damage theory]? It goes without saying that, for the most part, people in the besieged city were damaged by irregular eating and drinking and by excessive toil. Owing to two or three months of going hungry in the morning and eating their fill at night, rising and sleeping irregularly, and suffering from cold and heat due to being homeless, their stomach *qi* had long been exhausted. [Suddenly] eating excessively one day [as after the lifting of a siege] will have the effect of damaging people; and if, furthermore, treatment is inappropriate, then there is no doubt they will die. It was not only in Daliang [i.e., Kaifeng] that things were this way. Further back, during the Zhenyou and Xingding eras [1213–1222], [cities] like Dongping, like Taiyuan, and like Fengxiang were all the same in the illness and death they suffered after their sieges were lifted. In what I personally saw when I was in Daliang, there were some [physicians] who would effuse [the patients'] exterior (*biaofa* 表發); some who would press (*tui* 推) them with croton seed; some who would purge (*xia* 下) them with *Qi*-Restraining Decoction. Suddenly [their condition] would change to chest-bind or jaundice, and when they further purged (*xia*) them with Chest-Sinking Decoction or Pill and Virgate Wormwood Decoction, there were none who did not die. For it had not been Cold Damage in the first place, but because of mistakes of treatment it changed to resemble the symptoms of true Cold Damage; this was all the fault of the medicines.[104]

---

104 Li Gao, *Nei wai shang bian huo lun*, 8–9. It is important to note, since Li Gao is easy to misread here, that he is not talking about the effects of famine. Famine occurred in the Kaifeng siege, but at a

Here, the symptoms Li does specifically name are, as he sees it, the result of the treatments themselves. Thus presumably they cannot have preceded treatment: we are not learning what original symptoms these doctors were trying to treat. Yet in telling us how doctors were *treating*, Li is actually giving us clues as to what they *saw*. By itself, the fact that Li Gao is disputing a diagnosis of Cold Damage Disorder would tell us that the doctors were reaching that diagnosis, which would imply that the disease involved high fever. Some of his treatment notes imply no more than that. Both "Effuse the exterior," pointing to induced sweating to reduce fever, and "Purge them with *Qi*-Restraining Decoction" confirm high fever, and the latter was common in treatment of Cold Damage, as the first example of the formula comes from the Han-dynasty text that pioneered the Cold Damage category. But "press [*tui* 推] them with croton seed" may tell us more. The fundamental meaning of *tui* is "push" or "press," which tells us little since it is not a standard medical term, unlike *xia* for "purge." The known use of croton seed (not only in China) as an extremely vigorous purgative might suggest "purge" for *tui* too. But it would be strange for Li Gao to use the typical *xia* both for purging with *Qi*-Restraining Decoction and further on for purging with Chest-Sinking Decoction and Wormwood Virgate Decoction as well, and midway insert the very atypical *tui* for purging with croton. Why not simply "purged (*xia*) them with croton seed or *Qi*-Restraining Decoction" instead? Now *tui* can also mean "massage," and at this point it becomes intriguing that the fourth application of croton seed listed, in the modern *Practical Dictionary of Chinese Medicine*, is to induce a sore to rupture and discharge pus.[105]

The *Practical Dictionary* is a recent authority, of course. Were similar uses of croton known in and before Li Gao's own time? A digital search of Song and Jin medical texts for the term *badou* 巴豆, "croton seed," reveals—amidst a mountain of prescriptions involving croton as a purgative—a number of relevant mentions. The *Materia Medica Sorted by Syndrome* (*Zhenglei bencao* 證類本草) of Tang Shenwei 唐慎微 (fl. 1086–1094), published and republished between 1083 and 1116 in Northern Song but again in a Jin-period edition in the Taihe era (1201–1208), twenty-some years before the Kaifeng epidemic, tells us that croton seed can be used for "blade wounds where [flow of] pus or blood is inhibited"

---

much later stage, many months after the period in which Li Gao places the epidemic, as we know from the siege narrative of Liu Qi (*Guiqian zhi*, 11.126, lines 11–15, and 11.127, line 1). Li Gao is talking about *irregular* eating and drinking, irregular sleep, and excessive and irregular labour. Li Gao's "Internal Damage" medical theory was much concerned with both internal deficit (as may come from not eating enough) and surplus (as may come from eating too much), and here he is pointing, where food is the issue, to the irregular alternation of deficit with surplus. Months later, after the siege had been resumed and continued for months, both Liu Qi and the official history report residents eating saddles, leather boxes, their clothing, their own or other people's children, and each other. Nothing resembling this had yet occurred during the fairly short initial siege, which Li Gao tells us had lasted "half a month" before it was lifted, but which the official history places at ten or eleven days, and during which it appears the population was largely able to subsist on previously stored food—and perhaps initially even more able, after its numbers had been reduced by as much as a million.

105 Wiseman and Feng, *A Practical Dictionary of Chinese Medicine* (1998–2012), entry for *badou* 巴豆, item 4. Neither this very extensive entry on croton seed nor the particular item on its use to rupture sores and draw pus is found in the English-language print editions of the same dictionary: see Wiseman and Feng, *A Practical Dictionary* (2014).

(*jinchuang nongxue bu li* 金瘡膿血不利), and further on that it "discharges pus, resolves swelling-toxin, [...] treats malign sores" (*painong xiao zhongdu* [...] *zhi ecang* 排膿消腫毒... 治惡瘡).[106] Tang does not specify that the use is topical in these cases (though surely for sword wounds it would be), but later sources are more informative. An anonymous Northern Song work preserved in the Daoist canon prescribes a salve including croton seed to be applied (*tie* 貼, literally "stuck") onto haemorrhoids and refreshed each day; "when it reaches the sixth or seventh day, do not use painting it on (*tu* 塗) [any longer]; [instead] use pressing (*cui* 摧) the drug onto those that have not yet broken."[107] Haemorrhoids are obviously a special sort of sore, and expressing pus is not the object here; but the reference to "pressing" is intriguing, especially given the similarity of *cui* 摧 in both orthography and sound to Li Gao's *tui* 推; and the notable point is the topical use of croton (mixed with other ingredients) to break a sore. Chen Yan (1131–1189), in a work compiled in 1174, offers a salve of many ingredients, including croton seed, to "remove the nucleus from purple-black sores": the sore is to be pricked with a fine needle and the salve applied to the puncture-point. "The next day, press/push (*ji* 擠) on the sore; you will obtain (*you* 有) three ounces of black, foul-smelling pus and blood."[108] Li Xun's *Tested Prescriptions for Back Abscesses, Collected* (*Jiyan beiju fang* 集驗背疽方), dated 1196, similarly offers a multi-ingredient salve incorporating seven croton seeds and recommends that the physician "rub/massage (*ca* 擦) the drug onto the sore."[109]

In both of these last two examples, the use of verbs for rubbing or pressing again compares nicely to Li Gao's *tui*. Among Jin-period works, the *Treatise on Preserving Life according to Pathomechanisms and Suitabilities of the [Six Climactic] Qi of the "Basic Questions"*[110] (*Suwen bingji qiyi baoming lun* 素問病機氣宜保命集) of Liu Wansu prescribes a mixture of ingredients to be shaped into a "spindle" (*dingzi* 錠子) for direct application "to treat malign sores with dead flesh and to expel pus (*zhi echuang you sirou zhe ji zhui nong* 治惡瘡有死肉者及追膿)"; the ingredients again are multiple, but three croton seeds are to be mixed with a tenth of an ounce of each of five other components, so croton certainly appears quantitatively dominant.[111] Elsewhere in the same work, Liu recommends a mixture of croton with realgar—one bean of the former to a tenth of an ounce of the latter, so croton again dominates in volume and weight—"to treat all sores that contain bad flesh that cannot be eliminated (*zhi zhu chuang you erou bu neng qu zhe* 治諸瘡有惡肉不能去者)," with the note to "put a little onto the bad flesh, and it will depart of itself."[112] A "spindle" recurs in the *Confucian Service of Kin* of Zhang Congzheng 張從正 (1156–1228), where it is shaped out of six ingredients mixed with honey; later individual "cakes" or wafers (*bingzi* 餅子) are cut from the spindle and stuck (like stick-

---

106 Tang Tianwei, *Zhenglei bencao*, 14:3a–b. (*Zhongguo jiben gujiku* citation 14:571.)

107 Jijiu xianfang, 9:642.

108 Chen Yan, *Sanyin jiyi bingzheng fang lun*, 15:24a.

109 Li Xun, *Jiyan beiju*, 6a.

110 That is, the *Suwen* 素問 or "Basic Questions" section of the *Inner Canon of the Yellow Emperor*, *Huangdi neijing* 黃帝內經. I am grateful to Stephen Boyanton for his translation of the title.

111 Liu Wansu, *Suwen bingji qiyi baoming ji*, j. *xia*,下: 69–70.

112 Liu Wansu, *Suwen bingji qiyi baoming ji*, j. *xia*,下:70.

ing-plasters?) to each individual sore.[113] The honey is clearly a simple vehicle to make the other ingredients cohere, and these comprise forty-nine croton seeds to a half-ounce of one ingredient and tenth-ounce each of the other four, so once again croton dominates.

It might have been natural for Li Gao to refer to formulas like the last three in a generalizing way as "croton seed," since it considerably outweighs and outbulks its companion ingredients; but can one also find cases of croton seed used alone, or nearly alone? The *Skillful Prescriptions for General Aid, Sorted by Syndrome* (*Leizheng puji benshi fang* 類證普濟本事方) of Xu Shuwei 許叔微 (1079–1154) lists a prescription for "welling-abscesses and flat-abscesses that already have an eye but have not yet produced pus": a mixture of croton seed and fermented soybeans is to be formed into a wafer (*bingzi* 餅子) "the size of a mouse dropping"; this is to be applied to the mouth of the sore, and while "for a moment it will be unavoidably painful, after a good while the pus will come out."[114] The fermented soybeans outnumber the croton seed fourteen to one; but while fermented soybeans are a known medicinal when taken orally, they are unusual in a topical treatment, so it seems likely that here they are merely the vehicle enabling application of a single active ingredient, croton seed. A pediatric work of 1156 offers a salve for expelling pus and blood from malign sores (*echuang* 惡瘡): the two ingredients are twenty beans of croton seed and one ounce of lead oxide.[115] Elsewhere in Zhang Congzheng's *Confucian Service*, he offers a "Prescription for a Medicine for Bursting Dead Flesh," (*hui sirou yaofang* 潰死肉藥方) requiring the clinician to add graded quantities of croton seed to "cooked rice ends" (*chuifan jian* 炊飯尖) for varying degrees of strength, the mixture to be "put into the sore" (*na chuang* 納瘡); "when what is expelled is clear water, the bad flesh is not yet exhausted; once it expels red water, then the bad flesh is exhausted" (*zhui ye qingshui qi e'rou wei jin zhi zhui chishui shi e'rou jin* 追也清水其惡肉未盡至追出赤水是惡肉盡).[116] The cooked rice can only be a vehicle to deliver the croton; here again, croton seed seems the sole active ingredient.

The examples given here are illustrative, not exhaustive; but they constitute clear evidence that middle-period prescription texts, all preceding Li Gao's encounter with the epidemic at Kaifeng, recognized topical application of formulas including croton seed, and sometimes croton seed alone (or almost alone in appropriate vehicles) for treatment of purulent sores and in particular to expel pus and other fluids from them; and that they often deployed a variety of terms meaning "press, push, rub" (*cui* 摧, *ji* 擠, *ca* 擦) to describe how such formulas should be applied, closely paralleling Li Gao's *tui* 推, "press." Recall also that the late Southern Song or Yuan author of the *Pasture-Director's Collection* had used one of these very verbs, *ca* 擦, for "rubbing" a horse's *geda* to make it burst. All this leaves little room for doubt, I think, that in writing "some pressed them with croton seed," Li Gao meant "some rubbed them with croton seed formulas to expel pus from their sores." We have already seen that two of Li Gao's own stu-

---

113 Zhang Congzheng, *Rumen shiqin*, 15:188.

114 Xu Shuwei, *Leizheng puji benshi fang*, 6:13b–14a.

115 *Xiaoer weisheng zongwei lun fang*, 20:278.

116 Zhang Congzheng, *Rumen shiqin*, 15:188–89.

dents were prominent in bringing *geda* into epidemic discourse in the Yuan. In his surviving works Li Gao, unlike those students, never used the term *geda*, but an informed reading of his account of other doctors' treatments compels the inference that those doctors were treating a condition of high fever displaying large purulent lumps; and on my argument, these were the buboes of *Yersinia pestis*.

Conclusion

For a long time in Europe and North America, neither the field of Chinese studies nor that of Mongolian studies was very kind to William McNeill's 1976 proposal for an East Asian origin of the western Eurasian Black Death. As recently as six years ago, the leading economic historian of premodern China in the USA, Richard von Glahn, wrote that "The absence of evidence for a bubonic plague pandemic in China in the mid-fourteenth century militates strongly against McNeill's assertion that the mortality experienced in China was linked to the Black Death."[117] A leading Mongolist had declared, a few years before, that there is "no demonstrable mass outbreak [of] plague in China."[118] I found both judgments premature before I undertook the new research in this article, and find them more so now. To the former assertion, one might reply that until first Fan Xingzhun and later Cao Shuji and Li Yushang, hardly anyone had *looked* for evidence; Fan, Cao, and Li looked and claimed to have found it, without much impact till recently—perhaps because they published in Chinese?—on the European and American fields. Here I have sharpened, systematized, and expanded upon their evidence to support an argument for a first outbreak of plague in the thirteenth century. To the second declaration, one might respond that "demonstrable" is a prematurely high bar when research had as yet neither gone very far nor used all extant primary evidence. More recently Timothy Brook, having earlier cast doubt on the possibility of Chinese plague in the period of the European Black Death,[119] has developed a much more sympathetic take on the question for both the Yuan and (as we have seen) the seventeenth century, particularly in his important book *The Great State*. I see Brook's work as a welcome sign that the field of Chinese history has become more open to the possibility that the Second Pandemic included China, and that collaborative work and exchange on the issue has become a real possibility among historians of China, as Green and others were pioneers in making collaborative trans-Afro-Eurasian plague history possible.[120]

---

117 Von Glahn, *Economic History of China* (2016), 545n90.

118 Buell, "Qubilai and the Rats" (2012), 129.

119 Brook, *The Troubled Empire* (2010), 65–67. Brook followed Ole Benedictow, *The Black Death*, in finding the distance from China or Mongolia to the European jumping-off point for plague in the Crimea an insuperable obstacle to transmission by human or animal movement, and thus to any connection between Chinese epidemics and the European Black Death. His position, at that point, on the possibility of Chinese plague in the seventeenth century was less clear, but he seemed willing to entertain it (see 251).

120 Brook, *The Great State* (2020), 53–75 for the Yuan and 243–44 for the 1640s, where he supplies contemporary descriptions that could hardly *not* be plague. Like Monica Green, and indeed strongly influenced by her work, Brook places the likely site of the plague's thirteenth-century "Big Bang"

But von Glahn's "absence of evidence," if less accurate now than it might have been then, still points to a real issue that calls for exploration. If the argument of the present study is correct, evidence *has* survived in the changing symptom descriptions in medical texts, and has simply needed to be recognized. But on a larger scale, one cannot deny the absence in China of the kind of record or longterm cultural memory of *subcontinental-scale epidemic disaster* that one finds in European memory of the Black Death. To my eye, the likeliest explanation at this point is that Chinese historiography and cultural memory largely folded a (to some degree) similar epidemic experience in the thirteenth century into the historically well-understood, periodically expected, and (in China) recurrent human catastrophe of dynastic change and accompanying war, with consequent famine, disease, and general social disorder seen as natural concomitants.

If framing massive epidemic losses in this way was something like a common cultural tendency of those experiencing and recording the events of this period, what sort of evidence might one still expect or ought one still to look for, and what sort of finding would count as evidence? That is: *If something like the Black Death had occurred in China, how would it be reflected in the particular kinds of sources that Jin and Yuan China were likely to produce and that were likely to survive?* One would look first of all, surely, for large-scale population loss at the Jin–Yuan transition—and in fact, such evidence abounds and is largely accepted in the field.[121] But what more circumstantial kinds of testimony would one

---

in Kyrgyzstan (72–73), though unlike Green he does not explicitly associate it with the Mongol conquest of Qara Khitai. I should note that Brook's concluding "China was thus not likely the origin of the Black Death" (73), though it seems to be responding partly to my previous work, does not actually contradict my own position there or here, since I do not consider the Gansu corridor (site of the Tangut Xia state) or the Qinghai–Tibet plateau in the thirteenth century to have been "China" any more than Qara Khitai was, whatever modern maps may say about the former. On the historical difficulties posed by the too free use of the words "China" and "Chinese" in periods where their application is questionable, see Andrew Chittick's excellent *The Jiankang Empire* (2020), 9–35 and very abundantly *passim*.

121 In work that many consider the most authoritative treatment of Chinese population history now available, Wu Songdi estimates the population of all of Song-Jin China at its early thirteenth-century height at as high as 140 million, and the population of the roughly corresponding (actually somewhat larger) area under the Yuan in 1290 as 75 million: a stunning loss of 43 percent. Notice that the latter figure reflects fifty or so years of peace since the Mongol conquest of Jin, which had presumably allowed time for the population to recover, implying even greater loss in the crucial conquest period from the 1210s to 1234—though there is no way to estimate how much of this loss was from epidemic as opposed to war, since the wars of the conquest were themselves quite destructive, at least in the north: Wu, *Liao Song Jin Yuan shi qi*, 621, from *Zhongguo renkou shi* (2000). That the loss was heavily concentrated in North China (by 1290 the Yuan had also conquered South China)—that is, in the former Jin territories with which Li Gao's testimony is concerned—is clear from Wu's examination of region-by-region populations in North China for Jin and Yuan respectively: see 405 (for Henan), 414–15 (for Shandong), 425 (for Guanzhong), 443 (for Hebei), 450 (for Hedong), 456 for Yannan (an exception to general decline through being the region of the Yuan capital city), and 463 for Daibei. For relatively early work in English, one may compare Ping-ti Ho's estimate of the population of Song-Jin China (that is, north and south combined) as being in the area of 110,000,000 for the entire Chinese world during the late twelfth and early thirteenth centuries (significantly lower than Wu's estimates, though Ho's detailed figures could actually be read as implying 120 to 150 million) to his earlier estimate of 65,000,000 for

expect to find? The quantity and wide variety of sources in which Black Death evidence survives in Europe are utterly unmatched in Jin-period China. Yuan Haowen kept and published a journal of the Kaifeng siege—he seems to have been present throughout—but tantalizingly, that book did not survive past the eighteenth century.[122] It is worth stressing again the point I have already made with respect to Li Gao's nearly lone testimony: how consequential the loss of *a single book* may be for historical understanding; and in China books, through being written or printed invariably on *paper*, were probably much more vulnerable to destruction than the largely parchment books and archival documents of the European fourteenth century. We have a (*post facto*) eyewitness account of the Kaifeng siege from another author, Liu Qi, who entirely leaves out the epidemic; but the evidence is overwhelming that Liu fled the city for the entire epidemic period—and who would want to admit to that, and mention the million dead he had escaped being one of?[123]

Yet not only contingencies like these have produced the relative absence of evidence. In a separate work, I hope to explore the ways in which Chinese sources of the period put systematic evidentiary obstacles in the way of research on plague because epidemics lay outside the topics that Jin or Yuan gentlemen of the *shidafu* stratum—the authors of the majority of our sources—could envision as proper to mention in formal genres of writing. Yuan Haowen, we have seen, indirectly confirms Li Gao's mentions of two epidemics in other cities besides Kaifeng in the 1210s to 1220s, though perhaps only because he needs to find things to praise in the lives of two subjects of epitaphs, a praise genre; but Yuan's presence in Kaifeng during the Mongol siege in 1232–1233[124] has left us no mention of epidemic in

---

early Ming: encompassing two transitions, that from Jin to Yuan and that from Yuan to Ming, but in any case amounting to staggering loss from the early thirteenth to the late fourteenth century: Ho, "An Estimate" (1970), especially 52; and Ho, *Studies on the Population of China* (1959), 9. In 1969, Dwight Perkins, too, found devastating loss concentrated in North China between Song-Jin and Yuan: *Agricultural Development in China* (1969), 196–98. In 2010, Timothy Brook (*The Troubled Empire*, 43) appears to accept significant population loss associated with the Mongol conquests, though perhaps not as dramatic: a decline from over 100 million in Jin-Song to between 70 and 90 million in 1290. In 2016, Richard von Glahn, describing North China after the Yuan conquest, notes that "the agricultural economy was in a shambles and North China had suffered severe population losses. The registered population of North China declined by two-thirds between the Jin census of 1209 and the inaugural Ming census of 1393": *The Economic History of China* (2016), 279. There have of course been skeptics, as well: in 1987, Hans Bielenstein saw Chinese population history as a steady upward curve from about 700 to 800 CE on, with a jump upward to a much steeper slope of the curve about 1700: "Chinese Historical Demography," 72, 85, 154–56. Still, the current consensus in the field is that the Jin–Yuan transition saw profound population loss in North China. Major social reorganization and wholesale elite replacement founded on demographic disaster is certainly the impression one receives from Jinping Wang's very important recent study, *In the Wake of the Mongols* (2018).

122 Chan, "*Renchen zabian* yu *Jinshi* shiyuan" (1990), 188. See also his *Historiography of the Chin Dynasty* (1970), Part 2: 67–119.

123 See Hymes, "A Tale of Two Sieges" (2021), especially 332–43.

124 Yuan even mentions the Kaifeng epidemic itself in one book preface, to another of Li Gao's works, the *Treatise on Spleen and Stomach* (*Piwei lun* 脾胃論): "In the past, when we encountered the disaster of *renchen* (1232), and within fifty or sixty days those who perished from the damage done by eating, drinking, and exhaustion approached a million, everyone said that they had perished from Cold Damage. It was only later, when I saw [Li Gao's] treatise on distinguishing inner and

the many hundreds of poems for which he is most famous, let alone any trace there of the hundreds of thousands of epidemic deaths he must have personally witnessed or known of in 1232. Did elites like Yuan largely escape the outbreak, and were the commoner dead who were trundled out in piles (as Li Gao tells us) through the city gates in wagons simply beneath a gentleman's literary notice? Interestingly, we know that while Li Gao's patients included many gentlemen, his practice extended to ordinary people as well. Were his eye and writing brush open to the sufferings of a wider span of society not just because he was a physician, but because he was a physician with regular contact across class lines?

Disease in general and epidemic disease in particular are mostly non-topics in Jin writings, which are universally the work of elites—except in the writings of physicians, the sources I have worked with here. There is a global topic here for future comparative exploration: do the literate recorders of different societies record and remember parallel experiences of mass epidemic death in different ways, and if so, why? How do either the differing nature of written sources, their differential survivability, or, in a larger way, differing cultural resources with which to process such experiences, determine what the historian gets to see and to know? Timothy Brook has made an important initial stab at such a question in his comparison of British and Chinese responses to sixteenth- and seventeenth-century epidemics (in this instance leaving the question of the identity of the Chinese disease[s] open)—though, in that period, the Chinese sources are far from as silent as in Jin and Yuan.[125] Monica Green and Nahyan Fancy have shown that the 1258 Mongol siege of Baghdad was accompanied by an epidemic outbreak that was almost certainly plague (buboes were unmistakably mentioned), yet historical memory of this was erased by the fourteenth century when the western Asian component of the Black Death arrived in force; vague awareness of an epidemic in 1258 was swamped by the memory of the death and destruction of the Mongol siege itself and by more recent and more widespread plague.[126] Citing Alfred Crosby, who has characterized American historical memory as having virtually "forgotten" the 1918 flu pandemic that overlapped with the last stages of the First World War,[127] Fancy and Green ask "Is there something about the combination of epidemics and the trauma of war that produces a special kind of amnesia?"[128]

This jibes well with my suggestion that the experience of plague in Jin–Yuan China was folded into the overall experience of destructive conquest and dynastic change. But I have generally been conceiving that conflation as a virtually society-wide act of psychological and historiographic processing. Yet "society" did not write Chinese history. If we move to a smaller, individual-level scale and consider just the particular people in

---

outer damage and on the damage of eating, drinking, and exhaustion, that I realized the mistakes of common physicians." See *Yuan Haowen wen biannian jiaozhu*, ed. Di, 1018–19. This is the only place in Yuan's extensive surviving works where he mentions an epidemic that he personally lived through and that left around a million dead. But this preface was a favour to his close acquaintance Li Gao, who occasionally treated his illnesses too.

125 Brook, "Comparative Pandemics" (2020).

126 Fancy and Green, "Plague and the Fall of Baghdad" (2021).

127 Crosby, *America's Forgotten Pandemic* (2003).

128 Fancy and Green, "Plague and the Fall of Baghdad" (2021), 177.

North China in the early-to-middle thirteenth century who *could have* recorded plague for us, we might look at the example of Yuan Haowen. The Jin officeholding and examination elite, or the elements of it that survived the repeated Mongol attacks of the 1210s and 1220s, seems to have moved virtually *en masse* to the (recently shifted) capital at Kaifeng and its region in response to just those attacks. Yuan Haowen was one such man.

Yuan was in the capital because he had fled conquest and death that had already lasted, sporadically, twenty years or so; he was also an officer of the Jin state, in which office-holding was more central to elite identity than in its southern Chinese counterpart the Song. Yuan next lived through a siege of more than a year (if he did not, like Liu Qi, flee the capital for a time), interrupted early on by a temporary lifting and a devastating epidemic, which we will posit that he witnessed. The resumption of war shortly after the end of the epidemic brought the resumption too of devastating artillery attacks (perhaps largely by catapult) on the capital's city wall by the Mongols, to which the defenders inside the walls responded with deafening and terrifying bomb-throwing and fire-throwing weaponry of their own. This was not the first known use of large-scale gunpowder weaponry in war, by more than a century,[129] but it was surely the first that Yuan or his contemporaries had ever experienced. Much later in that more than year-long siege came a famine that (again) saw the people of the capital eating each other and each other's children, and wagons again trundling corpses out through the city gates, this time of the starved. When the siege finally ended in a Mongol sack of the city, Yuan and his fellow Jin officeholders were frog-marched in lines out of the city, initially they knew not whither, and he (along with others) spent the next couple of years more or less imprisoned in Shandong. In the meantime, they had seen the imperial family and much of the personnel of the court executed by a usurper even before the Mongols sacked the city; and by 1234, they knew that the Jin state had finally fallen and that the emperor—who had first fled the capital with a personal army—had killed himself when the Mongols took the city he had fled to.

Yuan knew that the state he had spent part of his life working for, and the community of officials, scholars, and writers who had constituted his network and shared in defining his identity in adult life, was scattered and—at least as a collectivity—largely gone. Should we expect that his experience of all this would have focused him closely on an epidemic that—like everything else that had happened—had failed to kill him? For those of his social stratum, the experience of the 1230s to 1240s was surely one of general and manifold loss of identity, status, and place, in favour of invaders of incomprehensible language and mores who seemed to have arisen from nowhere in the previous two decades and whom, at this stage, Yuan's ilk really did see as barbarians at best. But he and a small number of his literate and literarily inclined fellows were the only people who could have written the plague history we now wish we had. Is it that surprising if (as it appears) they did not?[130]

---

129 See Andrade, *The Gunpowder Age* (2016), 39, on the siege of the same city of Kaifeng by Jin invaders in 1127: "the Jin used gunpowder arrows and huge catapults hurling gunpowder bombs. The Song countered with gunpowder arrows, gunpowder bombs, thunderbolt bombs, and a weapon called the "molten metal bomb." See also pages 39–40 on the 1132 siege of De'an, when individual-level hand-borne flamethrowing "fire-lances" were used by the defending Song side.

130 There is, of course, the matter of Yuan's journal of the siege, already mentioned. If in that work,

They were the only ones, that is, except for that other stratum of literate practitioners, occupational physicians: *voilà* Li Gao. Yet even on the special turf of physicians' writings, as I have argued, one must conceive one's question carefully. Again, given a long and continuous previous history of epidemic diseases in China and the well-established field of Cold Damage medical theory that had arisen almost a thousand years before to cope with them, one should not expect physicians of the Jin and Yuan to report "Here is a terrible new disease!" with an accompanying detailed symptomatic description that one will instantly recognize as plague. Rather, my question has had to be, again: Given the predispositions and previous history of Chinese medical theory and practice, do disease descriptions across the Song–Jin–Yuan–Ming span, including attention to certain symptoms, change in ways that suggest an encounter with a new phenomenon in the period? They do; and the relatively sudden incorporation of a large purulent lump, often called *geda* (almost a brand new term in medical usage), into a number of categories or constructions of febrile and often fatal epidemic disease that were already established within previous medical discourse, is very much the response one might expect from middle-period Chinese physicians upon the entry into China of what *we now* would see as the new disease of plague.

Jin–Yuan physicians encompassed the entry of plague by absorbing it into pre-existing epidemic conceptions—while yet marking something importantly new about it through the addition of one symptom, the *geda*. This was a different approach, it seems, than doctors of the Mediterranean world took. And yet it is also striking that one disease name devised much later by some medical authors during the Ming–Qing transition of the seventeenth century, *geda wen*, "*geda* epidemic," is precisely parallel both semantically and in syntactic construction to the name "bubonic plague," attested in English no later than 1713.[131] Here, for once, Chinese and Europeans processed disease in at least the same terms, if not otherwise in the same way.

Back to Global Plague Genetics

I began by acknowledging the strong plausibility of Monica Green's recent reconstruction of the possible origin and trans-Eurasian paths of thirteenth- and fourteenth-century plague, based on a combination of up-to-date genetic evidence and historical work, and the enormous care for evidence and argument that her work displays. It is very possible that Green has got things entirely right, and that (for instance) future ancient-DNA evidence will support her picture. Yet I think (again) that reasons may remain for

---

unlike Liu Qi, he offered an account of the epidemic, then in later years he may well have felt that he had said his piece on that, was done with it, and wished to move on from the entire siege experience.

131 The *Oxford English Dictionary* gives the earliest date for the compound "bubonic plague" as 1803: "J. R. Manley *Inaug. Diss. Yellow Fever* 12 Bubonic plague would become epidemic in the same manner, whether in the torrid latitude of Gambia, or in the frozen regions of Zembla." Yet I think we can infer its presence no later than 1713, and probably a good deal earlier, judging by the suggestion of an already established usage in this entry for "bubonic": "1713 in T. Creech tr. *Lucretius Of Nature of Things* (new ed.) II. 778 The modern Physicians believe, that true Plagues, or those Infections, at least, which they call Bubonick, are disseminated by Contagion only."

entertaining my older argument for the 1206–1227 invasion of Xia—or indeed other possibilities that no one has yet identified, or a mix of possibilities—rather than the 1216–1218 invasion of Qara Khitai—as the Mongols' first encounter(s) with the plague bacillus, from which ultimately the Chinese experience traced here would follow, as well as and the later experiences of those in western Asia, North Africa, and Europe during the fourteenth century, along with later plague encounters in other Eurasian and African locations. The reasons are both empirical—including some bits of possible evidence touched on in passing in this article—and methodological.

On the empirical side, there is the question of timing, and of bringing Chinese evidence into line with the 1216–1218 Mongol conquest of the Qara Khitai state. Yuan Haowen's epitaph testimony to a siege-associated epidemic in the region of Taiyuan (one of the three cities Li Gao specifically mentions), when combined with the evidence on Mongol movements from chronicle sources, seems to place the beginning of the relevant siege in 1216, specifically in its second Chinese month, and its lifting some time in the ensuing ten months—but probably not very late in that span, since the Mongols returned and attacked the city afresh in the twelfth month.[132] (Bear in mind that Li Gao places each of his epidemics after the "lifting" of the respective siege.) This sits uncomfortably close in time to Chinggis Khan's commencement of his assault on Qara Khitai in 1216; in fact, Michal Biran's narrative would imply that the campaign against Qara Khitai *followed* the Mongols' departure from Taiyuan.[133] Even if the Qara Khitai campaign actually preceded or was simultaneous with the Taiyuan siege, to bring the Qara Khitai conquest into causal relation to things happening in the Taiyuan region—to suppose, that is, that Mongols transported the bacillus from the Tian Shan region to the North China plain in time to spawn an epidemic in Taiyuan—one might need to imagine transfers of Mongol troops back to Taiyuan from Kyrgyzstan in the midst of Chinggis's Qara Khitai campaign, covering a distance of more than two thousand miles. We don't know such movements didn't happen, but a need to posit them would be awkward. Taiyuan was finally taken in 1218, so even if that final siege (which was never "lifted," in the sense that Li Gao's term [*jiewei* 解圍] usually means, but simply carried through to completion) was the epidemic trigger, the events remain uncomfortably close in time to the Qara Khitai campaign.

Now, perhaps Li Gao's testimony misleads, and there was no relation between the epidemic at Taiyuan and those at the other cities he mentions, including Kaifeng, even though he judged them as parallel phenomena. Yet Li Gao's identified sieges were not even the earliest point at which sources point to an association between the Mongols and epidemics. As we have seen in Chart 2.1, the first such mention falls in 1211, when the chief minister of the Jin state, in the aftermath of the first Mongol incursions into

---

132 The relevant sources are *Jinshi* (Zhonghua shuju edition), 14:316, line 14; 14:322, line 6; 15:332, line 8; 15:333, line 7; and Yuan Haowen, "Guangwei jiangjun Guo jun mubiao," *Yuan Yishan wenji jiaobu zhong* 中:1011–12; but see the discussion in Hymes, "A Tale of Two Sieges," 302–5.

133 See Michal Biran, *The Empire of the Qara Khitai* (2005), 83–84. I have not so far been able to recover from Biran's sources a month, let alone day, for the assault on Qara Khitai; but her narrative tells us that "in 1216, soon after he had concluded his war with the Jin, Chinggis Khan sent his famous general Jebe to [then usurper of Qara Khitai rule] Güchüllug." The "war with the Jin" referred to in this instance is the wide-ranging campaign in North China that included the siege on Taiyuan.

Jin-controlled North China, is recorded to have reassured his ruler to this effect: "I have heard that the men and horses of the [Mongols], not suited to the water and land [in which they find themselves], are experiencing pestilence."[134] This evidence is vague, of course, and does not specify any particular disease; yet it is striking that it comes from a Mongolian, not Chinese source, the *Secret History of the Mongols*. Again, not all epidemics need be the same disease, and Occam's Razor is an unreliable standard for research and argument in history; but this source was one of the first that sent me, in my earlier work, hunting for possible references to plague in Chinese sources. There may not be, in sum, a perfect fit between the earliest mentions of Mongol-associated epidemic in or near China, on the one hand, and the hypothesis of an origin in the Qara Khitai conquest, on the other. History being the fuzziest of sciences, we cannot expect a perfect fit; but perhaps there is wiggle room just here for an account of the origin of thirteenth-century Central Asian / Chinese plague centred on the conquest of Xia—or possibly an account that entertains multiple "first" Mongol contacts with the bacillus. Mongol attacks on Xia began in 1205 and recurred in 1206 and 1209, as well as in 1217 (midway through the Qara Khitai campaign but far away from it) and 1224 before the final campaign of conquest in 1226–1227.[135]

Methodologically, as I know Monica Green would agree,[136] we cannot directly infer the past geographic distribution of strains of the plague bacillus from the present distribution—even though it is currently the best evidence we have—and thus infer where it was possible for which historical human population to contact which strain. It is anything but hard to imagine that the pre-polytomy strains now confined to the Tian Shan region were once much more widely distributed—perhaps, indeed, all the way from the Tian Shan to Gansu and the Qinghai Lake region, where now only later strains have (so far) been found. In fact, further searching might even still locate surviving pre-polytomy strains in those more eastern areas; but more probably, the post-polytomy strains now found there may simply have displaced the preceding pre-polytomy strains through dying-off and replacement of successive rodent populations one by another. (In much the same way, the plague strains responsible for the First Pandemic, the Justinianic Plague, appear to have vanished not just from that one region but from the face of the earth.) Green has used the very best genetic evidence now available to us, and is to be commended for constructing both a plausible and, frankly, a magnificent historical picture out of it. But anything closer to certainty about where Mongol forces first encountered plague (assuming, as both Green and I have concluded, that they did) may need to await the discovery of ancient DNA evidence from excavated human or rodent remains. Green has done the basic trans-Eurasian–African genetic work on which all future work

---

134 Bao, ed., *Yuanchao mishi* (2005), 173; see also *The Secret History of the Mongols*, ed. and trans. Cleaves (1982), 184 and 186.

135 Hymes, "Epilogue: A Hypothesis" (2014), 286.

136 In fact Green, a rigorously scrupulous scholar, says so: "The living descendants of Branch 0 are currently found in or near the Tian Shan range at the modern border between the Uyghur Autonomous Province and Kyrgyzstan; *this is not in and of itself proof of the medieval whereabouts of Branch 0*, but it provides data from which further inquiries could build." See Green, "The Four Black Deaths" (2020), 1625 (emphasis mine).

on the Second Pandemic must build. In the meantime I have tried to ground the Chinese component of that picture on a firmer historical basis, by showing that Chinese physicians' understanding of disease could allow them to absorb a new disease encounter into their categories without always explicitly recognizing it as new, and (except in the remarkable case of Li Gao) without associating it, as I have done through its striking timing, with the advent of the Mongols.

Bibliography

Primary Sources

Bao, Sitao 鮑思陶, ed. *Yuanchao mishi*. Ji'nan: Qilu shushe, 2005.

Chen, Shigong 陳實功. *Waike zhengzong* 外科正宗). Ming Wanli era (1573–1620) woodblock edition. (Found in *Zhongguo jiben gujiku*.)

Chen, Yan 陳言. *Sanyin jiyi bingzheng fang lun* 三因極一病證方論. Siku quanshu zhenben, fourth collection. Taipei: Taiwan shangwu yinshu guan, 1973

Cleaves. *See The Secret History of the Mongols*.

Deng, Jiezheng 鄧介正 and He, Wenlong, eds. *Simu anji ji* 司牧安驥集. Beijjing: Zhongguo Nongye chubanshe, 2001.

Dongyuan shizhong yishu 東垣十種醫書.Taipei: Shunfeng chubanshe, 1968.

Dongyuan yiji 東垣醫集. Edited by Ding Guangdi 丁光 and Wang Kui 王魁. Beijing: Renmin Weisheng chubanshe, 1992.

Jia, Sidao 賈似道. *Cuzhi jing* 促織經. Ming Yimen guangdu 夷門廣牘 edition. (Found in *Zhongguo jiben gujiku*.)

——. *Qiuqiong pu* 秋蟲譜. Ming Jiajing woodblock edition. (Found in *Zhongguo jiben gujiku*.)

Jijiu xianfang 急救仙方. In *Zhengtong Daozang* 正統道藏 1186, 26:599–658.

Jinshi. Edited by Tuotuo (1313–1355) et al. Zhonghua shuju edition. Beijing: Zhonghua shuju, 1975.

Jin-Yuan si da jia yixue quanshu 金元四大家醫學全書. Tianjin: Tianjin kexue jishu chubanshe, 1994.

Jin-Yuan si da jia yixue quanshu 金元四大家醫學全書. Edited by Wang Jun 王軍 et al. Tianjin: Tianjin kexue jishu chubanshe, 1994.

Li, Gao 李杲. *Nei wai shang bian huo lun* 內外傷辨惑論. In *Dongyuan yiji*, 1–49.

Li, Gao. *Huofa jiyao* 活法機要. In *Dongyuan yiji*, 335–72. Also included in *Jin-Yuan si da jia yixue quanshu*.

Li, Xun 李迅. *Jiyan beiju fang* 集驗背疽方. Siku quanshu edition. Taipei: Shangwu yinshu guan, 1983.

Liu, Qi 劉祁. *Guiqian zhi*. Collated and corrected by Cui Wenyin 崔文印. Beijing: Zhonghua shuju, 1983.

Liu, Wansu 劉完素. *Suwen bingji qiyi baoming ji* 素問病機氣宜保命集. Congshu jicheng edition. Beijing: Zhonghua shuju, 1985.

Luo, Tianyi 羅天益. *Dongyuan shixiao fang* 東垣試效方. Zhongguo yixue zhenben re-edition of Yuan edition. Shanghai: Zhongyi kexue jishu chubanshe, 1984.

Luo, Tianyi. *Weisheng baojian* 衛生寶鑒. Beijing: Zhonghua shuju, 1991.

Meng, Yuanlao 孟元老. *Dongjing menghua lu* 東京夢華錄. Wenyuange siku quanshu edition. Taipei: Taiwan shangwu yinshu guan, [1983].

Menggu mishi. *See* Bao, Sitao.

Pang, Anshi 龐安時. *Shanghan zong bing lun* 傷寒總病論. Congshu jicheng edition. Beijing: Zhonghua shuju, 1985.

Qi, Dezhi 齊德之. *Waike jingyi* 外科精義. Congshu jicheng edition. Beijing: Zhonghua shuju, 1985.

The Secret History of the Mongols: For the First Time Done into English out of the Original Tongue and Provided with an Exegetical Commentary. Vol. 1. Edited and translated by Francis Woodman Cleaves. Cambridge, MA: Harvard University Press, 1982.

Shen, Zhou 沈周. *Kezuo xinwen* 客座新聞. Qing manuscript edition, 11 j. (Found in *Zhongguo jiben gujiku*.)

[Sinongsi 司農司]. *Nongsang jiyao* 農桑輯要. Siku quanshu zhenben, special collection. Taibei: Shangwu yinshu guan, 1975

Sun, Simiao 孫思邈. *Yinhai jingwei* 銀海精微. Qing Zhihetang 致和堂 woodblock edition. (Published in Zhongguo jiben gujiku.)

Tang, Shenwei 唐慎微. [*Chongxiu Zhenghe Jingshi zhenglei beiyong*] *Zhenglei bencao* (重修政和經史證類備用)證類本草. Sibu congkan facsimile of Jin Taihe (泰和, 1201–1208) Huiming (晦明) edition. (Found in *Zhongguo jiben gujiku*.)

Tao, Zongyi 陶宗儀. *Chuogeng lu* 輟耕錄 (1366). Beijing: Zhonghua shuju, 1959.

Uibang yuch'wi 醫方類聚 (Compiled by decree of King Sejong, 1447). Seoul: Kŭmyŏng Ch'ulp'ansa, 1977–.

Wang, Guan 江瓘. *Mingyi leian* 名醫類案. Siku quanshu zhenben, sixth collection. Taipei: Taiwan shangwu yinshu guan, 1976.

Wang, Haogu. *Yilei yuanrong* 醫壘元戎. Siku quanshu zhenben, fourth collection. Taipei: Taiwan shangwu yinshu guan, 1973

Wang, Haogu / Li Gao, *Cishi nanzhi* 此事難知. Congshu jicheng edition. Beijing: Zhonghua shuju, 1991.

Wang, Kentang 王肯堂. *Zhengzhi zhunsheng* 證治准繩. Sikuquanshu edition. Taipei: Shangwu yinshu guan, 1983.

Wenyuange Siku quanshu dianziban (Electronic database of the *Siku quanshu*). 3rd ed. Hong Kong: Zhongwen daxue and Digital Publishing, 2007.

Wu, Qian 吳謙. *Yizong quanlan* 醫宗金鑒. Qing Qianlong era (1736–1795) Wuyingdian 武英殿 woodblock edition. (Published in *Zhongguo jiben dujiku*.)

Wu, Youxing 吳有性. *Wenyi lun* 瘟疫論. Sikuquanshu edition. Taipei: Shangwu yinshu guan, 1983.

Xiaoer weisheng zongwei lun fang 小兒衛生總微論方. Siku quanshu jiben gujiku, sixth collection. Taipei: Shangwu yinshu guan, 1976.

Xu, Guozhen 許國禎. *Yuyaoyuan fang* 御藥院方. Japanese Kanshō era Seishidō 精思堂 woodblock edition. (Published in *Zhongguo jiben gujiku*.)

Xu, Shuwei 許叔微. *Leizheng puji benshi fang* 類證普濟本事方. Sikuquanshu zhenben, fifth collection. Taipei: Shangwu yinshu guan, 1974.

Yifang leiju 醫方類聚. Edited by Zhejiang sheng zhongyi yanjiusuo 浙江省中醫研究所 and Huzhou zhongyiyuan 湖州中醫院.) Beijing: Renmin weisheng chubanshe, 1981.

Yu, Chang 喻昌. *Shanglun pian* 尚論篇. Siku quanshu zhenben, second collection. Taipei: Shangwu yinshu guan, 1971.

Yuan chao bi shi. See *The Secret History of the Mongols*.

Yuan, Haowen. *Yuan Haowen wen biannian jiaozhu*. Edited by Baoxin Di 狄寶心. Beijing: Zhonghua shuju, 2012.

——. *Yuan Yishan wenji jiaobu* 元遺山文集校補. Edited by Zhou Liesun 周烈孫 and Wang Bin 王斌. Chengdu: BaShu shushe, 2012.

Zhang, Congzheng 張從正. *Rumen shiqin* 儒門事親 (Congshu jicheng edition). Beijing: Zhonghua shuju, 1991.

Zhang, Jiebin 張介賓. *Jingyue quanshu* 景岳全書. Siku quanshu zhenben, tenth collection. Taipei: Shangwu yinshuguan, 1980.

Zhongguo jiben gujiku 中國基本古籍庫. In *Airusheng* 愛如生 (*Erudition*). Airusheng shuzihua jishu yanjiu zhongxin.

Zhou, Boqi 周伯琦. *Hucong ji* 扈從集. In *Wenyuange Siku quanshu dianziban*. 3rd ed. Hong Kong: Zhongwen daxue and Digital Publishing, 2007.

Zhu, Su. *Puji fang* 普濟方. Siku quanshu zhenben, twelfth collection. Taipei: Shang wu yinshu guan, 1982.

Secondary Sources

Andrade, Tonio. *The Gunpowder Age*. Princeton: Princeton University Press, 2016.

Anon. "The Plague. The Antitoxin Serum." *British Medical Journal* 1.1884 (February 6, 1897): 357a–359a.

Barker, Hannah. "Laying the Corpses to Rest: Grain, Embargoes, and *Yersinia pestis* in the Black Sea, 1346–48." *Speculum* 96, no. 1 (January 2021): 97–126.

Benedict, Carol. *Bubonic Plague in Nineteenth-Century China*. Stanford: Stanford University Press, 1996.

Benedictow, Ole. *The Black Death, 1346–1353: The Complete History*. Woodbridge: Boydell, 2004.

Bielenstein, Hans. "Chinese Historical Demography, A.D. 2–1982." *Bulletin of the Museum of Far Eastern Antiquities* 59 (1987): 1–185.

Biran, Michal. *The Empire of the Qara Khitai in Eurasian History: Between China and the Islamic World*. Cambridge: Cambridge University Press, 2005.

Brook, Timothy. "Comparative Pandemics: The Tudor–Stuart and Wanli–Chongzhen Years of Pestilence, 1567–1666." *Journal of Global History* 15, no. 3 (2020): 363–79.

——. *The Great State: China and the World*. London: Profile, 2020.

——. *The Troubled Empire: China in the Yuan and Ming Dynasties*. Cambridge, MA: Belknap, 2010.

Buell, Paul. "Qubilai and the Rats," *Sudhoffs Archiv* 96, no. 2 (2012): 127–44.

Cao, Shuji 曹树基. "Dili huanjing yu Song-Yuan shidai de chuanranbing 地理环境与宋元时代的传染病." *Lishi yu dili* 历史与地理 12 (1995): 183–92.

——. "Shuyi liuxing yu Huabei shehui de bianqian, 1580–1644 鼠疫流行與華北社會的變遷, 1580–1644," *Lishi yanjiu* 歷史研究 1 (1997): 17–32.

Cao, Shuji 曹树基 and Li Yushang 李玉尚. *Shuyi: Zhanzheng yu heping—Zhonnguo de huanjing yu shehui bianqian, 1230–1960 nian* 鼠疫：战争与和平：中国的环境与社会变迁（1230–1960 年）. Ji'nan: Zhongguo huabao chubanshe, 2006.

Chan, Hok-lam (Chen Xuelin 陳學霖). *The Historiography of the Chin Dynasty: Three Studies*. Wiesbaden: Steiner, 1970.

——. "*Renchen zabian* yu *Jinshi* shiyuan 壬辰雜編與金史史源," *Guoli Taiwan daxue lishi xuebao* 國立臺灣大學歷史學報 15 (1990): 185–95.

Chittick, Andrew. *The Jiankang Empire in Chinese and World History*. Oxford: Oxford University Press, 2020.

Crosby, Alfred W. *America's Forgotten Pandemic: The Influenza of 1918*. 2nd ed. New York: Cambridge University Press, 2003.

Cui, Yujun et al. "Historical Variations in Mutation Rate in an Epidemic Pathogen, *Yersinia pestis*." *Proceedings of the National Academy of Sciences* 110, no. 2 (2013): 577–82. Prepublished December 27, 2012.

Cunningham, Andrew. "Transforming Plague: The Laboratory and the Identity of Infectious

Disease." In *The Laboratory Revolution in Medicine*, edited by Andrew Cunningham and Perry Williams, 209–44. Cambridge: Cambridge University Press, 1992.

Dunstan, Helen. "The Late Ming Epidemics: A Preliminary Survey." *Ch'ing shih wen-t'i* 3, no. 3 (1975): 1–59.

Fan, Xingzhun 范行准. *Zhongguo yishi shilue* 中國醫學史略. Beijing: Zhongguo guji chu-banshe, 1986.

Fancy, Nahyan. "Knowing the Signs of Disease: Plague in the Arabic Medical Commentaries between the First and Second Pandemics." In *Death and Disease in the Medieval and Early Modern World*, edited by Lori Jones and Nükhet Varlık, 35–66. York: York University Press, 2022.

Fancy, Nahyan and Monica H. Green. "Plague and the Fall of Baghdad (1258)." *Medical History* 65, no. 2 (2021): 157–77.

Fong, Mary H. "Tang Tomb Murals Reviewed in the Light of Tang Texts on Painting." *Artibus Asiae* 45 (1984): 35–72.

Green, Monica H. "The Four Black Deaths." *The American Historical Review* 125, no. 5 (December 2020): 1601–31.

Hanson, Marta E. "Late Imperial Epidemiology, Part 1: Historiography of the History of Disease in China, 1870s to 1970s," and "Late Imperial Epidemiology, Part 2: New Material and Conceptual Methods from the 1980s to 2010s." In *The Routledge Handbook of Chinese Medicine*, edited by Vivienne Lo and Michael Stanley-Baker, 245–62 and 263–81 respectively. London: Routledge, 2021.

——. *Speaking of Epidemics in Chinese Medicine: Disease and the Geographic Imagination in Late Imperial China*. Abingdon: Routledge, 2011.

Ho, Ping-Ti. "An Estimate of the Total Population of Sung-Chin China." *Études Song / Sung Studies* 1 (1970): 33–52.

——. *Studies on the Population of China, 1368–1953*. Cambridge, MA: Harvard University Press, 1959.

Horrox, Rosemary, ed. *The Black Death*. Manchester: Manchester University Press, 1994.

Hymes, Robert. "A Tale of Two Sieges: Liu Qi, Li Gao, and Epidemics in the Jin–Yuan Transition." *Journal of Song Yuan Studies* 50 (2021): 295–363.

——. "Continuous Transformation? A Reconsideration of Andrew Cunningham on the Historical 'Identity' of Plague, and Possible Implications for the History of Medicine." Paper presented at the Pennsylvania State University. April, 2016.

——. "Epilogue: A Hypothesis on the East Asian Beginnings of the *Yersinia pestis* Polytomy." *The Medieval Globe* 1 (2014): 285–308. Reprinted as *Pandemic Disease in the Medieval World: Rethinking the Black Death*, edited by Monica H. Green, with Carol Symes. Bradford and Kalamazoo: Arc Medieval [Humanities] Press, 2015.

Liu, Yan. *Healing with Poisons: Potent Medicines in Medieval China*. Seattle: University of Washington Press, 2021.

McNeill, William. *Plagues and Peoples*. New York: Anchor, 1976.

Mitchell, Piers. "Retrospective Diagnosis and the Use of Historical Texts for Investigating Disease in the Past." *International Journal of Paleopathology* 1 (2011): 81–88.

Nikoforov, Vladimir V. et al. "Plague: Clinics, Diagnosis, and Treatment." In *Yersinia Pestis: Retrospective and Perspective*, edited by Ruifu Yang and Andrey Anisimov, 293–312. Dordrecht: Springer, 2016.

The Oxford English Dictionary. 3rd ed. Oxford: Oxford University Press, 2020.

Perkins, Dwight. *Agricultural Development in China, 1368–1968*. Chicago: Aldine, 1969.

Pfister, Rodo. "Üble Kerne unter der Haut: Neu erschlossene medizinische Quellen, zur Beulenpest im frühmittelalterlichen China." In *Pest! Eine Spurensuche*, edited by Stefan

Leenen, Sandra Maus, and Doreen Molders, 64–73. LWL-Museum für Archäologie, Westfälisches Landesmuseum Herne. Darmstadt: Wissenschaftliche Buchgesellschaft, 2019.

Royer, Katherine. "The Blind Men and the Elephant: Imperial Medicine, Medieval Historians, and the Role of Rats in the Historiography of Plague." In *Medicine and Colonialism: Historical Perspectives in India and South Africa*, edited by Poonam Balsa, 99–110. London: Pickering and Chatto, 2014.

Spyrou, Maria S. et al. "Analysis of 3800-Year-Old *Yersinia pestis* Genomes Suggests Bronze Age Origin for Bubonic Plague." *Nature Communications* 9, no. 1 (June 8, 2018): 2234.

Spyrou, Maria S. et al. "The Source of the Black Death in Fourteenth-Century Central Eurasia." *Nature* 606 (2022): 718–24.

Twitchett, Denis. "Population and Pestilence in T'ang China." In *Studia Sino-Mongolica: Festschrift für Herbert Franke,* edited by Wolfgang Bauer, 35–68. Münchner ostasiatische Studien, 25. Wiesbaden: Steiner, 1979.

von Glahn, Richard. *The Economic History of China: From Antiquity to the Nineteenth Century.* Cambridge: Cambridge University Press, 2016.

Wang, Jinping. *In the Wake of the Mongols: The Making of a New Social Order in North China, 1200–1600*. Cambridge, MA: Harvard University Asia Center, 2018.

Wiseman, Nigel, and Feng, Ye. *A Practical Dictionary of Chinese Medicine.* 3rd ed. Taos: Paradigm, 2014.

——. *Practical Dictionary of Chinese Medicine (Chinese and English).* Phone-app version: Pleco Revision 1. Taos: Paradigm, 1998–2012.

Wu, Lien-teh et al. *Plague: A Manual for Medical and Public Health Workers.* Shanghai: Weishengshu National Quarantine Service, 1936.

Wu, Songdi 吳松弟. *Liao Song Jin Yuan shi qi*, vol. 3. of *Zhongguo renkou shi*, ed. Ge Jianxiong 葛剑雄. Shanghai: Fudan University Press, 2000.

Wu, Tianchi 吳天墀. *Xi Xia shi gao* 西夏史. Chengdu: Sichuan renmin chubanshe, 1983.

Yersin, Alexandre. "Sur la peste bubonique (sero-therapie)." *Annales de l'Institut Pasteur (Journal de Microbiologie)* 11 (1897): 81–93.

Appendix 2.1

References for Table 2.2

1. 1090. Throat Closure (*houbi* 喉閉) (Recorded 1090–1099): Pang Anshi, *Shanghan*, 3:75.
2. 1138–1149. (No name); "presentation similar to Thunder Head (*leitou* 雷頭)" (recorded 1156–1161): quoted in *Shiyuan's Proper and Effective Prescriptions* (*Shiyuan duanxiao fang* 施圜端效方), which in turn is quoted in the nineteenth-century Korean compilation *Uibang yuch'wi*, reprinted in China in 1982 as *Yifang leiju* (179:419).
3. Before 1186. Big Head (*datou* 大頭) and Thunder Head Wind (*leitou feng* 雷頭風) (recorded 1186; no specific dated event mentioned): Liu Wansu *Suwen bingji qi yi baoming ji, xia* 下: 136–37.
4. 1202. Seasonal Toxin (*shidu* 時毒); Big Head Heaven-Current (*datou tianxing* 大頭天行) (recorded 1266): Luo Tianyi, *Dongyuan Shixiao fang*, 9:1a.
5. 1206–1207. *Nue* (intermittent high fevers) and "miasmic pestilence" (recorded 1228): Zhang Congzheng, *Rumen shiqin*, 1:75–81.
6. 1213–1222. Unnamed epidemics in Taiyuan, Dongping, and Fengxiang, reported to be similar to the 1232 Kaifeng siege epidemic (recorded 1247): Li Gao, *Nei wai shang bian huo lun*, 8–9.
7. Before 1228. Thunder Head (recorded 1228; no dated event mentioned): Zhang Congzheng *Rumen shiqin*, 4:330.
8. 1232. Kaifeng siege epidemic (recorded 1247). No disease name given; reportedly mistaken for Cold Damage: Li Gao, 8–9.
9. Before 1253. Throat Closure; Big Head; Thunder Head; Seasonal Qi (*shiqi* 時氣); Epidemic Qi (*yiqi* 疫氣) (recorded 1253; no dated event recorded): Wang Haogu, *Yilei yuanrong*, 4:4b.
10. Before 1264. Thunder Head (recorded 1264; no dated event mentioned): Wang Haogu/Li Gao, *Cishi nanzhi*, j. *xia*, 14b–15b.
11. Before 1267. Seasonal Toxin; Seasonal Disease (*shiji* 時疾); "in presentation similar to Thunder Head" (recorded in 1267; no dated event mentioned): Xu Guozhen, *Yuyaoyuan fang*, 7:11a (*Zhongguo jiben gujiku* citation 7:122).
12. Before 1281. Thunder Head Wind "presenting like Cold Damage" (recorded in 1281; no dated event mentioned): Luo Tianyi, *Weisheng bao jian*, 9:371–72.
13. Before 1281. Seasonal Toxin (recorded in 1281; no dated event recorded): Luo Tianyi, *Weisheng bao jian*, 9:373.
14. Before 1281. Seasonal Epidemic (*shiyi*) (recorded in 1281; no dated event mentioned): Luo Tianyi, *Weisheng bao jian*, 9:373.
15. ca. 1300 ("Yuan"). Seasonal Epidemic; Swelling Toxin (recorded ~1300; no dated event mentioned): *Shiyuan's Proper and Effective Prescriptions*, quoted in *Uibang yuch'wi. Yifang leiju*, 179:419.
16. Before 1335. Seasonal Toxin (recorded 1335; no dated event mentioned): Qi Dezhi, *Waike jingyi, shang* 上: 84–86.
17. Before 1335. Seasonal Toxin; Big Head Illness (recorded 1335; no dated event mentioned): Qi Dezhi, *Waike jingyi, xia* 下: 31.
18. Before 1406. Toxin Swelling; Swelling Toxin (*zhongdu* 腫毒); Seasonal Epidemic (recorded 1406; no dated event mentioned): Zhu Su, *Puji fang*, 279:1a–21a.
19. Before 1447. Swelling Toxin; Seasonal Epidemic (recorded 1447; no dated event mentioned): *Uibang yuch'wi*, reprinted as *Yifang leiju*, 179:419.

Robert Hymes (rph2@columbia.edu) is H. W. Carpentier Professor of Chinese History at Columbia University. His previous research has dealt mostly with the social and cultural history of the Song and Yuan dynasties in China, especially focused on local history, history of elites and elite-state relations, and history of religion, mostly in southern China. In those connections he is the author of two monographs, *Statesmen and Gentlemen: The Elite of Fu-chou, Chiang-hsi in Northern and Southern Sung* (1986) and *Way and Byway: Taoism, Local Religion, and Models of Divinity in Sung and Modern China* (2002); co-editor of the volume *Ordering the World: Approaches to State and Society in Sung China* (1993); and author of the chapter "Song Society and Social Change" in Volume 5, Part Two of *The Cambridge History of China* (2015). In collaboration with Anna Shields of Princeton University, he is currently undertaking a pair of conference volumes on the change from Tang to Song, growing out of the Conference on Tang-Song Transitions which they co-organized at Princeton in June, 2022. In 1997, he had attempted a research foray into the possibility of plague in Jin–Yuan China (moving into the unfamiliar territory of North China for the first time), but found the discoverable sources too sparse to support definite conclusions. In 2014, Monica Green and Carol Symes invited him to contribute, as a representative of East Asian history, an epilogue on plague in China to the inaugural volume of *The Medieval Globe*. In the meantime, the China field had been transformed by the emergence of massive digital databases of premodern Chinese sources; the invitation thus started him on a long-term inquiry into plague in middle-period China that has so far produced two further articles: "A Tale of Two Sieges" (2021) and the present article. The work on plague will continue.

Abstract In a previous contribution to *The Medieval Globe*, I proposed the hypothesis that certain epidemics reported in association with the Mongol invasion of China and adjacent states during the thirteenth century and after were plague, and perhaps the first historically recorded manifestation of the Second Pandemic. This article supports that hypothesis using evidence largely from Chinese medical texts of the eleventh through the eighteenth centuries, to show that these epidemics in North Chinese cities directly followed Mongol sieges, as reported by the thirteenth-century physician Li Gao (who witnessed one of them). In turn, they were followed (within twenty-five to fifty years) by the appearance of a brand new symptom in Chinese medical texts: a large purulent sore, called by a name almost new to Chinese medical discourse and entirely new in discourses on epidemic: *geda*, which I argue was the label applied to the bubo of plague. I show further that Li Gao's description of the treatments attempted by doctors during the siege epidemic of 1232, in the Jin-dynasty capital Kaifeng, strongly imply that the doctors were treating such large purulent sores; and that two of Li Gao's students were leaders in introducing the term *geda* to epidemic discourse in the decades that followed. What distinguished the response of Chinese physicians to plague from the response of their later European counterparts, I conclude, was that they largely registered its presence by incorporating a new symptom into older epidemic categories rather than by seeing it as a new disease. In a foreword and afterword I frame my work in the context of Monica H. Green's recent ambitious and highly persuasive picture of thirteenth-and fourteenth-century plague as a many-branched global phenomenon.

Keywords Black Death, bubonic plague, *Yersinia pestis*, Chinese medicine, Mongols, Li Gao, Yuan Haowen, *geda*, epidemic disease

PUTTING ASIA ON THE BLACK DEATH MAP

MONICA H. GREEN[*]

THE APPEARANCE OF Robert Hymes's essay, "Buboes in Thirteenth-Century China: Evidence from Chinese Medical Writings," brings *The Medieval Globe* back to its roots eight years ago. In 2014, Hymes presented his initial thoughts on how the then-emerging evolutionary history of the plague bacterium, *Yersinia pestis*, might relate to massively lethal epidemics in Jin-era northern China that seemed to be plague-like in their manifestations. Could plague's late medieval proliferation have started more than a century before the Black Death of the mid-fourteenth century, long known through documentation from western Asia, Europe, and North Africa? Could it have first struck, not in Europe or any landmasses adjacent to the Mediterranean, but East Asia?[1]

At the time, Hymes introduced his assessment as "a hypothesis." It is much more than a hypothesis now. It is at the center of a growing paradigm shift in how historians think about the semi-global experience of plague in the later Middle Ages and early modern period;[2] indeed, it has sparked an entire rethinking of how the field of medical history might move beyond stalled debates on whether modern disease categories can inform historical investigations. But as with all paradigm shifts, this one, too, is creating rifts in opinion. Just as Hymes's new essay was undergoing its final revisions, a study appeared in the science journal *Nature* claiming that the Big Bang—the sudden polytomy or profusion of *Y. pestis* into new ecological niches—had happened not in the thirteenth century, as Hymes (and others) postulated, but definitively in the early decades of the fourteenth century.[3]

Some tensions can be salubrious for a field, and I think this one ultimately will be. As they relate to Asia's history, the emerging debates in plague history are pushing investigators—historians and scientists alike—to think concretely about our questions, our methods, and our standards of proof (or at least, persuasion).[4] Hymes's 2014 essay took genetics seriously and asked how the hints it offered of a medieval Asian history of plague might be substantiated in insufficiently interrogated historical records. It is now time for genetics to do the same, taking Hymes's discoveries seriously and asking how "the biological archive" connects with the documentary evidence that plague was a compounding factor in the devastation that northern China endured in the first half of the thirteenth century.[5] Indeed, all of Asia likely merits investigation.

---

[*] My thanks to Professor Susan Einbinder, University of Connecticut at Storrs, for many fruitful conversations about plague's increasingly entangled histories.

[1] Hymes, "Epilogue: A Hypothesis" (2014).

[2] For a general assessment of studies to date, see Varlık, "Plague in the Mediterranean/Islamicate World" (2022).

[3] Spyrou et al., "Source of the Black Death" (2022).

[4] Green, "Out of the East" (2022).

[5] On the "biological archive" see Green, "The Four Black Deaths" (2020).

The present essay is intended to lay out the larger scene on which Hymes's arguments, as well as the new palaeogenetic evidence, should be set. To open ("Sketching
the Outlines of the Map"), I summarize the main developments in the field of plague
studies in the eight years since *Pandemic Disease in the Medieval World: Rethinking the
Black Death* appeared. Then, I argue that, to move forward in reconstructing plague's
history, it is necessary to do two things. First (Section 2, "Populating the Map: The Role
of aDNA in Reconstructing Plague's History"), it is necessary to admit that, with a disease as complex in its mechanisms and manifestations as plague (involving not simply
the microscopic pathogen itself but also arthropod vectors and rodent hosts, all of them
susceptible to the varying effects of climate), evidence from multiple disciplines must be
mobilized to document the disease's presence, symptoms, epidemiological trajectories,
and social impact. But it also necessary to recognize why results coming from different disciplinary perspectives might conflict, one reason being that they yield evidence
for only random parts of a very large puzzle. Resolution of that conflict is essential if,
in fact, all parties agree that disease phenomena have a material, living substrate—a
Great Chain of Being, if you will, of biological connections that are real even if we cannot
always document them. Then, in Section 3 ("Opening Our Eyes to an Invisible Past: Time
Travel in a Global Middle Ages"), I argue that adding insights from a modern biological
understanding of a disease *whose presence at particular historical times and places can
be proven* (aptly called a kind of time travel) does not negate or disparage evidence of
how the people of the past themselves understood what they were experiencing. Plague
was, for long stretches, invisible to human actors, and here we need to let the microbe
tell its story. But that story must, in the end, be compatible with the story we construct
from human sources. This is the biggest challenge in the field right now. In my conclusion ("Defining the Second Plague Pandemic"), I argue that the weight of seven hundred
years of historiography needs to be recognized and, when necessary, set aside. We have
more insight into the physical conditions of the past than ever before, and we can see the
linkages that allowed a microbial agent to affect so many landscapes—precisely what
we mean by "pandemic." A global approach, which emphasizes patterns and linkages, is
justified to investigate both the medieval pandemic's enormity and its uniqueness.

Sketching the Outlines of the Map

Hymes's present article, published in this volume, forms the third part of a trilogy. In his
2014 essay, he laid out his hypothesis that China's later medieval history of pandemics
could be correlated with a recent proposition coming from genetics. In 2013, biologists
Yujun Cui and colleagues proposed that a Big Bang in plague dissemination—the sudden
displacement of a single highly lethal strain of plague into new ecological niches, creating four unique lineages which shared the same common ancestor—had likely occurred
sometime in the century and a half prior to the Black Death's conventional starting date,
1346. Hymes described the testimony of a Jin-era physician, Li Gao (d. 1251), who was
not simply present during the siege and epidemic of 1232 in the Jin southern capital,
Kaifeng, but had apparently altered his thinking about epidemic diseases in the years
thereafter, devising what he called an Internal Damage theory to account for the new

symptoms he witnessed.[6] In a 2021 sequel, Hymes expanded this work by assembling a corpus of evidence (often from passing asides in texts never meant to tell epidemic stories) for the routes of Mongol troops through Jin territory and the timing of reported epidemics. He drilled down into one particular question when pondering how to assess the magnitude of this previously unnoticed testimony. Why, he asked, did two literate witnesses of the same devastating siege at Kaifeng reveal such a major discrepancy in their accounts: one describing tens of thousands of deaths in what was then northern China's largest city, the other giving no indication that an epidemic had even happened? The answer, Hymes suggested, is that one of the witnesses wasn't present: he had likely fled the city during the most devastating phase of the crisis. The other witness, Li Gao, called in one source a "National Physician" of the Jin, had not only stayed but, in later years, correlated his observations at Kaifeng with the epidemic aspects of several other sieges, based on the testimony of numerous high-status patients and colleagues whom he consulted.[7] By dissecting poems and epitaphs, career trajectories and personal motives, Hymes established a tight chronology of key informants who testified to the occurrence of epidemics at the times and places of several Mongol sieges.

In the present essay, Hymes returns to the larger questions that he had originally posed in 2014 but could not then resolve, as to why there appeared to be changing conceptions of disease in contemporary Chinese medical sources. Writing in 1995 and 2006 and drawing on a variety of such sources, scholars Cao Shuji and Li Yushang had argued for plague's presence in China well before the late Jin period.[8] Here, Hymes examines the evidence more closely, tightly constraining it chronologically and showing a pattern that Cao and Li missed. In the thirteenth century, plague was what we would today call an "emerging infectious disease," a disease not hitherto described nor having any standardized method of treatment. Physicians had to decide whether this disease (which was consistently identified as *epidemic*, occurring and then disappearing just as rapidly) could be shoehorned into older categories of disease or whether it required a categorical rethinking. Li, the physician who had witnessed the Kaifeng siege in 1232, would go on to develop a new field of medicine, Internal Damage theory, which for him explained the particular characteristics of the new disease better than the "Cold Damage disorder" which then dominated Jin-era medical thinking on epidemics. Most importantly, Hymes documents that the concept of *geda*—a term perhaps originally meaning "knot," and in medical contexts signifying a large and purulent sore (memorably described in one instance as a polo-ball-sized swelling)—suddenly became a specialized referent for the key distinguishing symptom of this new disease entity. Moreover, Hymes demonstrates that both the word and the concept stuck: *geda* continued to appear in Chinese medical writings for six hundred years. In other words, Hymes establishes not simply that this was a new disease in the thirteenth century, but that it *persisted* as a disease concept that physicians felt they needed to address in their medical writings and, from time to time, that they had to treat.

---

6 Hymes, "Epilogue: A Hypothesis" (2014).

7 Hymes, "A Tale of Two Sieges" (2021).

8 See the citations in Hymes, "Buboes in Thirteenth-Century China" (2022).

There are two reasons why Hymes's observations about Li Gao and the epidemics of Jin-era China have risen in importance. One is that, in 2020 and 2021, two related studies brought forth evidence of thirteenth-century Mongol sieges, in regions outside of China, that could also be connected to plague-like incidents, this time during the western campaigns undertaken by Hülegü in the late 1250s. Nahyan Fancy and I discovered evidence from historical chronicles that fiercely lethal epidemics, characterized by buboes and blood-spitting, had struck populations besieged by Mongol troops in western Iran, Iraq, and Syria. Even the troops, it seems, had been devastated by the outbreaks. In the writings of physicians (or, in one case, a hadith commentator who had had medical training), there was a pronounced contemporary shift in the detail with which plague (*ṭāʿūn*), a category that had been a part of Islamic theology and law since the seventh century, was described.[9] But it wasn't just the parallel circumstance that plague seemed tied to Mongol military activity; it was the fact that a particular *mechanism* of transmission was being postulated: grain supplies shipped from the foothills of the Tian Shan mountains to the plains of western Iran. Although Hymes has not yet established the mechanisms that might have moved plague eastward to China in the thirteenth century, his rigor in constructing a *biologically plausible* story of what happened in Jin-era China—taking into account social networks, rhetorical genres, symptom descriptions, and many other factors—has opened the door to asking whether parallel instances might correspond to other "events" in *Y. pestis*'s evolutionary history.

The other reason why Hymes's original hypothesis (which his current article now substantiates) is more important than ever is that there is now palaeogenetic proof that the Big Bang—the sudden geographic dispersal of *Yersinia pestis* that was postulated by Cui and colleagues in 2013, and that has been supported by all phylogenetic studies since then—did occur as predicted.[10] As Hymes and the other contributors to the inaugural issue of *The Medieval Globe* already noted in 2014, plague history has been in the midst of what could be called an "evolutionary" or "genetics turn" since the late 1990s. Studying the genome of the bacterium (first fully sequenced in 2001) allowed the structure of the organism's evolution to come into view. Building on the technical achievement of the retrieval in 2011 of *Y. pestis* DNA from two dated fourteenth-century burial sites in London,[11] Cui and colleagues proposed that a sudden divergence happened sometime in the century and a half before the Black Death, creating four new lineages of plague. They could not, however, confirm *where* it happened. In 2018 and 2020, my own research combined the phylogenetic analyses of 2013 with newer field ecological sur-

---

9 Green, "The Four Black Deaths" (2020); Fancy and Green, "Plague and the Fall of Baghdad" (2021); Fancy, "Knowing the Signs" (2022).

10 "Phylogenies" in evolutionary biology are postulated family trees of organisms or species. At the genomic level, phylogenies are postulated on the basis of shared genetic mutations within lineages or strains.

11 In 2016, I established that one of the four genomes sequenced by Bos et al., "A Draft Genome" (2011), had, in fact, come from a burial site outside of the East Smithfield Black Death Cemetery. It related to the second (known) wave of plague's arrival in England, the *pestis secunda*. On the significance of the phylogenetic reconfiguration of Lineage 1B to the story of plague's dissemination within Europe, see Green, "Out of the East" (2022).

veys published in 2017 to suggest that the "Ground Zero" of plague's late medieval proliferation was not the Tibetan Plateau (as had previously been proposed) but further to the northwest, in or near the Tian Shan mountain range that lies on the border between modern Kyrgyzstan and the Xinjiang Autonomous Province: the very region from which grain had been shipped in the 1250s, according to a Persian source. As I showed, the surviving strains of *Y. pestis* that are most closely related to the genomes retrieved from Black Death sites in Europe are mostly found in marmot populations in or near the Tian Shan: see Plate 3.1.[12]

Then, in June 2022, one of the world's leading scientific journals published a paper announcing the retrieval of *Yersinia pestis* genomes from a medieval gravesite in northern Kyrgyzstan.[13] A community of Church of the East (Nestorian) Christians had lived in a small village called Kara-Djigach and had been accustomed to honouring their dead with inscribed gravestones, most of which indicated date of death. In one particular year, in which there was a noticeable spike in the number of deaths, a handful of the inscriptions also indicated cause of death: eleven individuals had died of *mawtānā*, pestilence.[14] Materials collected by the archaeologists who originally excavated the site in the later nineteenth century had been dispersed to a variety of different museums in Russia and neighboring states. The new investigators were able to retrieve enough of the remains, extracting ancient DNA (aDNA) from the teeth of three individuals, to confirm that the pestilence of which the gravestones spoke was indeed *Yersinia pestis*. And not only was it plague, it was a strain (labelled BSK001/003 in Plate 3.1[15]) that seemed to fall on the phylogenetic tree right before the Big Bang, supporting earlier inferences that the Second Plague Pandemic, the medieval Black Death, originated in Central Asia.

---

12 Cui et al., "Historical Variations" (2013); Green, "Putting Africa on the Black Death Map" (2018) and "The Four Black Deaths" (2020), the latter including a supplementary file, "Marmots and Their Plague Strains."

13 Spyrou et al., "Source of the Black Death" (2022).

14 My thanks to Mark Dickens for help in confirming the total number of gravestones mentioning *mawtānā* (ten), one of which commemorated a husband and wife. See the Supplementary Information of Spyrou et al., "Source of the Black Death" (2022), for further details on this unique burial site.

15 See https://doi.org/10.1038/s41586-022-04800-3. The original caption reads in full: "**a**, Maximum likelihood phylogenetic tree, based on 2,441 genome-wide variant positions. The tree was constructed to indicate the genetic relationships between available 0.ANT genomes depicted on the map and BSK001/003. Modern branches were collapsed to enhance tree clarity (see Extended Data Fig. 8 for a full tree). **b**, Map depicting the geographical isolation locations of 0.ANT strains (Supplementary Table 21), which belong to the closest ancestral branching lineages to the Kara-Djigach strain. The map includes both whole-genome data (further specified as 0.ANT lineages 1, 2, 3 and 5) and PCR-genotyped isolates that are broadly defined as 0.ANT, belonging to any of the 4 lineages. For strains in which exact geographical coordinates were unavailable, locations were approximated according to their associated plague reservoirs. To aid visibility in overlapping symbols, a jitter option was implemented for plotting objects on the map. The map was created with QGIS v.3.22.1 (ref. 51) and uses Natural Earth vector map data from https://www.naturalearthdata.com/."

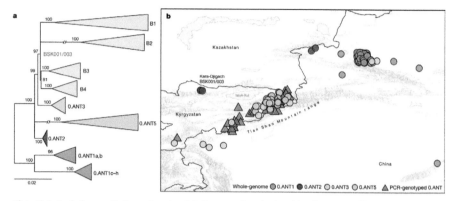

Plate 3.1. A phylogenetic tree showing (a) the genetic relationships between all genotyped 0.ANT genomes depicted on the map; and (b) BSK001/003, the strain of *Yersinia pestis* retrieved from the Christian cemetery of Kara-Djigach. Reproduced from Spyrou et al., "Source of the Black Death" (2022), fig. 4.

Within two weeks of its appearance, this study (published Open Access and subsidized by the Max Planck Institute, which had trained several of the researchers) had been directly accessed on the journal's website 206,000 times, garnering press coverage in all the world's major news outlets. But here's the rub. The authors proposed that the Big Bang most likely happened between 1308 and 1338, a full century after the Mongol expansion had begun. That the *Y. pestis* lineage immediately preceding the Big Bang was in existence at the latest by 1338 (the date of the documented plague outbreak in the Kyrgyzstan village from which the new plague DNA was retrieved) was already likely. The absolute *terminus ad quem* of the Big Bang was already established by the genomes retrieved from the dated Black Death Cemetery in London, i.e., 1348, since that genome is already two SNPs (single nucleotide polymorphisms) beyond the polytomy. The question, rather, is *how much earlier than 1338* could the Big Bang have happened? The Kara-Djigach genomes (labelled BSK001/003 on Plate 3.1 above) have all three of the SNPs that define the *Y. pestis* lineage that gave birth to the four documented post-polytomy lineages (postulated by Cui and colleagues in 2013), meaning that they are clearly part of the Big Bang phenomenon. Moreover, Spyrou and colleagues demonstrate that the Kara-Djigach genomes do not have any of the SNPs characteristic of the known post-polytomy lineages (Branches 1–4), meaning that the Kara-Djigach genomes do not constitute an early form of any lineage known today. Having made that determination, the authors then use computer programs (the results being visualized in a graph) to suggest that the Big Bang most likely happened after 1308 but before 1338, the established date of the epidemic in Kara-Djigach. In other words, they propose that *Y. pestis*'s late medieval emergence was a process *confined to the fourteenth century*, and not earlier.

Hymes's original argument, in 2014, did not hinge on any particular pre- or post-polytomy strain being involved in the Jin-era outbreaks. But my 2020 argument, based on parallel evidence of sieges in the 1250s which could have introduced Branch 1 (or its immediate ancestor) into western Asia, was tied to the Big Bang thesis. And Hymes's present article is now making an explicit argument for the *continuity* into the early modern period of thirteenth-century medical concepts—notably the adaptation of the term *geda* for buboes—and, by implication, the continuity of the disease. By 1308, the *terminus a quo* for the Black Death polytomy posited by Spyrou and colleagues, the Mongol campaigns of conquest, had long since ended. None of the evidence suggesting plague's presence in Jin China and mid-thirteenth-century Iran, nor the postulated circumstances (marmot habitat disruption followed by grain distribution) that may have given rise to plague's most marked re-emergence since the time of the First Plague Pandemic, was factored into their analysis, which in fact offered no *cause* for plague's alleged fourteenth-century emergence.[16] One hundred years of plague history, as tentatively reconstructed by Cui and colleagues, Hymes, Green, and Fancy, seems to have vanished.

Populating the Map: The Role of aDNA in Reconstructing Plague's History

Has the reconfiguration of Asia's plague history over the past eight years, as pioneered by historians and based on the findings of geneticists, been so insignificant that it can be superseded by a single computer-generated graph? A principal reason that palaeogenetics has established itself so quickly as a major arbiter in plague history is that it did indeed resolve a question at the heart of disease history generally. From the 1970s up through 2010, there was an ongoing debate, not so much among medical historians as among demographers, economic historians, and others, of what "really" caused the Black Death. The reasons for the debate need not be reviewed here, other than to say that it was the end result of skeptical stances feeding on themselves to the point of explanatory nihilism. The partial retrieval in 2010 of verifiable *Yersinia pestis* aDNA fragments, followed quickly by the retrieval of nearly complete genomes of the bacterium and demonstration of how little the medieval genome differed from modern isolates, effectively settled the question.[17] The Black Death was caused by *Yersinia pestis*.

However, in the decade since that question was settled, there has arisen a new one, namely: Is the successful retrieval of pathogen aDNA the *only* way to confirm the presence of a particular disease in a given time and place, or to establish other key turning points in plague's history? Here, an analogy with palaeopathology is important, since that discipline, too, is concerned with documenting and interpreting past experiences with disease.[18] Simply stated, palaeopathology can confidently identify the presence of certain diseases in material remains in those cases when the disease leaves pathognomonic signs in the bones or teeth. Thus leprosy, tuberculosis, syphilis, and a few other

---

16 Spyrou et al., "Source of the Black Death" (2022), 723: "the dynamics that triggered the bacterium's emergence in this region are unknown."

17 For a summary of the debates, see Varlık, *Plague and Empire* (2015), 91–94; on the early years of disputes about plague aDNA retrieval, see Little, "Plague Historians" (2011).

18 See Grauer, "A Century of Paleopathology" (2018), and Buikstra et al., "Introduction" (2017), on the principles and terminology that have developed in the field of palaeopathology over the past century.

diseases can be confidently diagnosed in given invduals that present with a certain con-stellation of skeletal lesions. Plague, in contrast, is such a quick killer that there is no bone remodelling in the few days it takes to kill its victim. For physical confirmation of plague in a given individual, palaeopathology must defer to palaeogenetics as the ulti-mate arbiter.

However, plague is not an "individual" disease. No infectious diseases are, of course, since the infecting organism must have come from somewhere. But whereas an individ-ual might harbour malarial parasites or leprosy or tubercular bacilli for years without engaging with another host or victim, plague is a "landscape" disease. As a historian of late antiquity, Peter Sarris, memorably put it:

> The evidence [coming from singular retrievals of plague aDNA] thus requires an imagina-tive and truly interdisciplinary response, less fixated with raw numbers [i.e., how many individuals can be shown to have *Y. pestis* in their bodies]. Certainly, if one were to find the body of an extraterrestrial buried on a Welsh hillside, one would hardly just dismiss it with words along the lines of: "Well, it is only *one* alien". One would want to know how it got there, and one would have to work on the assumption that the voyager probably had not travelled alone.[19]

The global evolutionary history of *Yersinia pestis* that geneticists have assembled in the past two decades—building, of course, on well over a century of plague field biology and laboratory analysis of the pathogen—tells us that we should never consider plague to be a voyager that travels alone. When plague shows up in human bodies, there is always a larger ecological process that explains how it got there.

The particular demands of plague—which for its long-term sustenance needs both rodent hosts and arthropod vectors (or, at the very least, soil conditions in which the bacterium can persist for short periods of time)—as well as its very distinctive epidemi-ological profile once it moves into susceptible mammalian hosts, allow us to distinguish it historically from other diseases known to cause epidemics. On this question, too, pal-aeogenetics has shown its considerable value to historical investigations, because a num-ber of other pathogens besides *Y. pestis* have now been successfully retrieved through the new technological methods of aDNA. Of most importance for differential diagnosis in situations of mass death is *Salmonella enterica enterica* Paratyphi C, or paratyphoid fever. A special, human-adapted serovar of *Salmonella* that, like plague, has been shown to have evolved within Eurasia, Paratyphi C likely emerged as a uniquely virulent strain sometime around the ninth century CE. It has been documented in a single individual from twelfth-century Norway, but also in mass burial sites in fourteenth-century Lübeck, Germany; sixteenth-century Mexico (an outbreak in Teposcolula-Yucundaa in the mid-1540s); and seventeenth-century Spain. It may have also been involved in a large-scale epidemic in Mexico in 1576, about thirty years after its first documented presence in New Spain. For the 1576 outbreak, detailed descriptions of the symptoms of what was called locally *cocoliztli* ("pestilence") come from contemporary witnesses, including Spanish friars, who listed among its symptoms "fevers, intense thirst, rapid pulse, jaun-dice, delirium, abscesses behind the ears, dysentery, and pain in the heart, chest, and

---

19 Sarris, "New Approaches" (2022), 339.

stomach."[20] Indigenous survivors focused on one symptom in particular: haemorrhage. The Nahua author of the *Anales de Tecamachalco* offers a particularly detailed description of the outbreak:

> [M]any people died: young people, married people, old people [men and women] and children. [...] In two or three days they died of hemorrhage, blood emerged from their noses, from the ears, from the eyes, from the anus. And women bled between their legs. And for us men, blood emerged from our members. Others died from diarrhea, which took them suddenly, they died quickly from this.[21]

Cocoliztli in early colonial Mexico gives us a useful example of the complexities involved in identifying past diseases for another reason. The fact that one epidemic is documented by aDNA (the one in 1545–1548) while the other is not (1576–1577) doesn't mean that we can know nothing about the latter; it means that we look for other indicators. First, the two outbreaks are separated by thirty years, meaning that some eyewitnesses from the first outbreak would still have been alive during the second. The fact that the same word, *cocoliztli* is used for both outbreaks; the fact that both outbreaks are depicted by similar iconographic signs; the fact that there are overlaps in symptom descriptions:[22] all these factors support as reasonable the inference that both epidemics were caused by *S. Paratyphi C*, whether because of its continued presence in Mexico from 1545 to 1576 or its reintroduction via the same contacts with Europe. Jennifer Scheper Hughes, who has recently offered a richly chronicled account of the survivance of the *pueblos de Indios* in the face of population loss and ruin, shows the cultural effects of this physical experience.

As Hymes reminds us, symptom descriptions are always filtered through a local, historically specific cultural lens, making their "translation" into universal somatic constants a perennial challenge. Still, we see nothing in the descriptions from 1576 Mexico of buboes or swellings of any kind. And Spanish observers in Mexico, who would have been well acquainted with the symptoms of plague by this point, described the Mexican disease as something they had never seen before.[23] The inferences we can make about the two epidemics in Mexico can also be applied to interpreting the disease's history in Europe, from which it came. We can expect that, in those cases where the disease struck in Europe, it would have produced similar, non-plague-like symptoms even if it also killed quickly and occasionally in large numbers. The exceptional presence of four mass graves in fourteenth-century Lübeck demonstrates how richly complicated disease history has become with the advent of a robust palaeogenetics, because they exemplify the ever-present challenge of data retrieval from long-decaying remains: two of the four gravesites (the larger ones) yielded no discernible pathogen aDNA at all, while the other two yielded not plague (as had been suspected) but Paratyphi C.[24]

---

20 Hughes, *Church of the Dead* (2021), 9.

21 Hughes, *Church of the Dead* (2021), 9.

22 For symptom descriptions of the 1545 outbreak, see Vågene et al., *"Salmonella enterica Genomes"* (2018), Supplementary Discussion 1.

23 Hughes, *Church of the Dead* (2021), 11. On Paratyphi C's history in Europe, see Green, "The Great Dying" (2021), 9–12.

24 Haller et al., "Mass Burial Genomics" (2021).

Here is where the comparison between plague and paratyphoid fever becomes especially important for our purposes: both diseases persist through "quiet phases" when they are not producing large-scale human mortality. But whereas plague's reservoir is rodents, paratyphoid fever's is most likely solely humans; it persists because, as with typhoid, certain individuals can be "carriers," keeping the bacterium alive (perhaps in their intestines, perhaps in bone lesions) while not being unduly debilitated by it. Whereas plague can be readily transmitted long distance by exploiting networks of grain or textile distribution, paratyphoid fever likely relies on individual human carriers transmitting the disease to local populations through fecally contaminated food or water. Plague outbreaks can be regional; paratyphoid fever outbreaks are likely to have been mostly local.[25] The epidemiological "landscapes" of the two diseases are completely different.

This is why the emphasis on networks matters in global approaches to the Middle Ages. Although more an umbrella of scholarly interests than a methodologically united field unto itself, these approaches have, more and more, been looking at intersections and patterns: at commodities or knowledge or concepts that travel and affect regions larger than those circumscribed by the narrowly limited political structures normally used for historical investigation. Moreover, the "biological archive" that the combined approaches of phylogenetics and palaeogenetics has opened allows analyses that move across not only geographical expanses but chronological ones, too.

While hugely consequential for studies of the premodern past, aDNA is a privileged kind of evidence. Not only is it rare, it can only be retrieved through highly controlled and expensive laboratory processes, and the many terabytes of sequence data can only be processed by high-throughput computers and with the specialized programs designed for this work. Even after all that labour and expense, it does not always produce impeccable data. Parts of the genome may be poorly attested, others may not be present at all. The data that is yielded may still be tremendously informative, especially when compared with modern genomes of much higher quality. But, as with many aspects of medieval research, the incompleteness of data matters. When attempting to answer the question of when plague's late medieval proliferation out of the Tian Shan region began, it should first of all be noted that Spyrou and colleagues were able to retrieve only about 93.5 percent of the postulated Kara-Djigach genomes. That means that there may be close to 30,000 positions (on a genome that usually runs to about 4.6 million base pairs in length) for which there is no data. This is relevant because although it is possible to be certain of most of the genomes' character, the missing 6.5 percent stands between us and confirming whether the genomes constitute a hitherto undocumented fifth branch in the post-polytomy tree postulated by Cui and colleagues or, as argued by Spyrou and colleagues, whether we have, against all odds, found the exact state of *Y. pestis* at the beginning of the most catastrophic pandemic in human history.[26]

---

25 If paratyphoid fever was the cause of the 1576–1577 outbreak in central Mexico, it may have found a mechanism of transmission thus far not documented in Europe. Hughes reports that "the viceroy Martín Enríquez wrote that it 'affects one town just a league away from another where it rages for a long while and later returns to it so that it appears as if it is a living thing and that it goes in search of towns so that none remain'": *Church of the Dead* (2021), 11.

26 Spyrou et al., "Source of the Black Death" (2022), achieved 93.5 percent coverage by adding

There is, moreover, another omission not directly addressed by Spyrou and colleagues. In estimating the evolutionary age of the Kara-Djigach strain, the researchers omitted one-third of the genomes they had selected for the study, including all the genomes of other *Y. pestis* strains found in the marmots of the Tian Shan, which make up the rest of Branch 0. (Again, see Plate 3.1.) Because of research on the Justinianic Plague genomes, which derive from the same main branch of *Y. pestis* but at an earlier evolutionary stage, we know that the marmot strains of Branch 0 likely originated about a millennium and a half before the Big Bang. Since marmots hibernate for half the year (likely putting *Y. pestis* into a non-infectious stasis), consideration of the particular rodent species hosting the bacterium is of some importance when assessing rates of mutation.[27] The calibration of Spyrou and colleagues, which captures only post-Big Bang *Y. pestis* strains (most of which have moved permanently out of marmot hosts), differs by a century from prior estimated ranges of the Big Bang's date, which had included the more slowly evolving Tian Shan strains.[28] In sum, while the Kara-Djigach study has successfully confirmed the presence of *Y. pestis* in 1338 at that specific site in Kyrgyzstan, the dating claims about the evolutionary "event" of the Big Bang must be bracketed for the time being as unverified. They will need to be assessed by further analytical and confirmatory studies.

In this limbo between disciplinary methods and their findings, where does the question of Asia's history with plague stand now? In its overleaping of previous studies devoted to the Big Bang's approximate date, the recent *Nature* paper ignores the question of how the evidence brought forward by Hymes (for China) and Green and Fancy (for western Asia) bears on the *interconnected* phenomena of the Second Plague Pandemic. Because it is a living organism, always needing to replicate, we know that plague existed *somewhere* in thirteenth-century Eurasia, because it had persisted there in some form or another since the Late Neolithic. Of course, it is possible that the episodes in Jin China and Ayyubid Baghdad and Syria, even if they can be attributed to *Yersinia pestis* as the assumed causal organism, are unrelated to each other and to the Big Bang. Because we do not yet have aDNA from either setting, we cannot say with certainty how or whether those episodes relate phylogenetically to what has been retrieved from Kara-Djigach in the fourteenth century.

But what if they are related? In 2020, I proposed that the "Four Black Deaths," the four lineages of *Y. pestis* created by the Big Bang, could all be tied to the environmental

---

together the genetic data from two individuals. This assumes, of course, that only one strain of *Y. pestis* was active in causing the Kara-Djigach outbreak.

27 Tang et al., "Plague Outbreak" (2022). Further evidence that marmots can hibernate carrying *Y. pestis* comes from the recent case of a herdsman who was infected in the middle of winter (which is not normally a season of plague infections) because he had dug a hibernating marmot out of its burrow; see Xi et al., "First Case Report" (2022).

28 Before the 2022 study by Spyrou and colleagues was submitted for peer review, Seguin-Orlando et al., "No Particular Genomic Features" (2021) had proposed a phylogenetic analysis of Branch 1 (the western Eurasian lineage produced by the Big Bang) which suggested that the lineage's manifold diversification occurred well before 1346, the date usually cited as the beginning of the Black Death's proliferation.

footprint created across Eurasia by the Mongol Empire. Take away any connections with the thirteenth century, and these causal links disappear. Leave them in consideration, and there are now two elephants in the room regarding plague's currently unaccounted-for century of history.

1. If highly lethal Second Pandemic *Y. pestis* strains *did* cause the outbreaks in thirteenth-century China, as well as in the Jazira (the region between the Tigris and Euphrates) and Syria, why did survivors' experience of massive mortality not produce Black Death-like testimonials? Why did the thirteenth century have neither the Boccaccios nor the Ibn al-Wardīs that the fourteenth century produced?[29] Why are we only learning about these episodes in the twenty-first century?

2. Why didn't the series of repeated, almost decadal, outbreaks that would characterize the experience of plague in western Asia, North Africa, and Europe from the 1360s on start a century earlier? In other words, why were the events in the 1220s and '30s described by Li Gao, and those in the 1250s described by Quṭb al-Dīn al-Shīrāzī (d. 1311) and Arabic chroniclers, followed, not by years of chaos, but by the *Pax Mongolica* or "Mongol Exchange," perhaps the most intense period of intercontinental exchange Eurasia had ever seen?

Let us take these questions in reverse order. Why was there no catastrophic, hemispheric Black Death immediately after these thirteenth-century outbreaks, and no repeating cycles of plague? First, the levels of *local* catastrophe described by Jin and Ayyubid sources are every bit as pronounced as any single outbreaks we see described in later, fourteenth-century sources. The process of focalization (embedding the disease in wild rodent populations, in which it can persist long-term) is different from the circumstances that spark epidemics in human communities. We are still uncertain of what processes plague would have needed to undergo to adapt to non-marmot ecologies, as plague must have done in order to become a regular source of outbreaks outside of the Tian Shan environment. At the very least, we have to assume that there must have been changes, not so much in the character of the pathogen, as in the flea and intermediate host ecology, in order for plague to be sustained outside of marmot-hosted environments.[30] At the moment, unfortunately, none of these processes of adaptation are documentable, since we have no evidence whatsoever of the insect vectors or early rodent hosts from this period. But as we will see in the next section, there is more evidence of

---

29 Although the *maqāma* of the Aleppan poet and historian Ibn al-Wardī (d. 1349) is not as universally famous as Giovanni Boccaccio's (d. 1375) *Decameron*, the former's poem in fact enjoyed immediate and long-standing circulation in the Islamicate world.

30 There is a common misconception that the Big Bang entailed some genetic shift in the virulence of *Yersinia pestis*. The Big Bang does not, however, refer to any documented genetic change in the organism. It is instead a signal that multiple clones of a single strain of *Y. pestis* (the pre-polytomy strain) moved into four new environments in which they then proceeded to thrive, creating descendants (with their own distinctive genetic changes) that have survived to the present day. It is fair to assume that the strains closest to the polytomy did not differ to any appreciable degree from their common ancestor.

continuity after the thirteenth century than discontinuity in terms of other evidence for plague's presence.

As for the lack of eloquent testimonials of catastrophic outbreaks in the thirteenth century (which may also account for their loss from the traditions of both Chinese and Islamicate world), Hymes has already addressed this question, as did Fancy and I.[31] Clearly, thirteenth-century physicians in both Jin China and Ayyubid Syria and Egypt reacted to a new, or newly visible, disease. Very close attention to the chronology of the evidence (for Hymes, the changing uses of *geda*; for Fancy and myself, the refined descriptions of *ṭā'ūn*, plague/bubo, and its clinical descriptions) allowed us to pinpoint when new disease awareness developed. Yet in both instances, historical memory around the events failed to gel. Describing the hardships that Yuan Haowen, Li Gao's colleague and fellow siege-survivor, had endured (gunpowder warfare, famine-induced cannibalism, imprisonment), Hymes notes that "he and a small number of his literate and literarily inclined fellows were the only people who could have written the plague history we now wish we had."[32] The chroniclers and physicians of Ayyubid Syria and Egypt may have escaped such personal hardships under the threat of the Mongols, but as Fancy and I observe, plague may not have seemed the most imminent concern in the midst of threatened conquest. Additionally, the constraints of different genres of writing, and different rhetorical objectives, may function to exclude epidemic disease as a topic of discussion.[33]

Bringing these observations back into consideration with the genetic evidence, we should also note that the accounts of thirteenth-century plague outbreaks newly assembled from documentary records provide something that the genetics narrative currently does not. Whatever date is assigned to the Big Bang (and it should be remembered that, biologically, that "bang" might have been a multi-decadal process), it must have had a precipitating cause. The assumption of both my "Four Black Deaths" thesis and that of Spyrou and colleagues is that the strains of *Y. pestis* now found in the marmots of the Tian Shan mountains and the adjacent Junggar Basin to the northeast have been there for centuries, perhaps throughout the entire Common Era. Aside from the Justinianic Plague in Antiquity, we do not have evidence that those reservoirs generated any other major diffusions of plague. The Big Bang and the ensuing Second Plague Pandemic are, with that one ancient exception, unprecedented.[34] Spyrou and colleagues offer no pre-

---

31 Hymes, "Buboes in Thirteenth-Century China" (2022), 8–9 and 44–49; Fancy and Green, "Plague and the Fall of Baghdad" (2021), 173–77.

32 Hymes, "Buboes in Thirteenth-Century China" (2022), 48. As Hymes observes in "A Tale of Two Sieges" (2021), 299–301,Yuan Haowen did record notes on the year of the siege, but they were lost by the eighteenth century.

33 My thanks to Susan Einbinder for this observation. Marien, "The Black Death" (2009), 27–28, itemizes the reasons why epidemic outbreaks might not be considered ennobling and therefore unlikely to be mentioned in accounts written, for the most part, to favor the experiences and perspectives of the upper classes.

34 Between the strains of *Yersinia pestis* involved in the proliferation that produced the Justinianic Plague—see Green, "When Numbers Don't Count" (2019) for a summary—and the divergence that produced the "twin" lineages, the pre-polytomy and 0.ANT3, the only surviving lineages are another set of twins, 0.ANT2 and 0.ANT5, which presumably took their origin sometime between

cipitating cause to account for plague's sudden eruption out of its long-term habitat. And since the Big Bang is an ecological displacement of plague, not a genetic mutation towards greater virulence or transmissibility, a fourteenth-century Big Bang stands, for the moment, unexplained.

If, however, we think of the Big Bang as *a process* instead of an event, we better understand what it represents. The dissemination of a pathogen is itself a network: every bacterium (or virion) is a link in the chain. We will never reconstruct those chains in each of their elements, but there is no need to do so. When patterns are found, when there is evidence of networks, these make biological connections plausible. As in the case of paratyphoid fever in Mexico, retrieval of pathogen aDNA from *each* outbreak of an on-going pandemic is not needed to make *reasonable inferences* of common causes and sustained transmission. Retrieval of aDNA from even just a few sites allows the creation of what we might call an inferential algorithm, where each additional kind of evidence (depending on its quality and consistency) builds confidence that we are getting close to reconstructing the world our historical subjects inhabited, just as Hughes was able to reconstruct the efforts of the *pueblos de Indios* of New Spain to find meaning in their suffering from *cocoliztli*. The work of the historian must go on, even if it must do so without reliance on the palaeogeneticist's standards of proof.

Table 3.1. Types of Evidence for the Historical Presence of Plague.

	Type of Evidence	Discipline	Utility
1	adjacent to plague-infected region	geography	Circumstantial: heightens likelihood that plague may have passed through the region
2	aDNA	genetics	Decisive: confirms plague's presence; for complete genomes, decisive for confirming evolutionary stage and suggestive for dating or directionality
3	surviving Second Plague Pandemic strain	genetics	Suggestive: indicates a possibility that the strain's ancestors may have inhabited the same ecosystem
4	written accounts—symptoms	history	Suggestive to decisive: depending on the level of detail, can be decisive in plague diagnosis
5	written accounts—swift, large-scale epidemics	history	Suggestive: few other known diseases produce as much mortality in as short an interval of time
6	disrupted ruling or social structures	history	Circumstantial: a clue that something is amiss, possibly due to sporadic epidemics

the ninth and twelfth centuries. These have been found only in or near the Tian Shan. On the still slim evidence for a possible pan-Eurasian plague pandemic in the eleventh century, see Ellenblum, *Collapse* (2012); I am not aware that this eleventh-century episode, if it was caused by *Yersinia pestis*, created enduring reservoirs.

	Type of Evidence	Discipline	Utility
7	linguistic (terminology) —oral or written lore	history anthropology	Suggestive: the existence of a social or medical category for a disease shows that it has meaning within the culture; meanings and referents can change
8	mass burials	archaeology	Suggestive: need to be distinguished from other possible causes (war, targeted violence, famine)
9	signs of abandonment	archaeology	Suggestive: can be multi-causal (famine, long-term climatic shifts, major earthquakes, war) and may show migration rather than absolute population loss
10	signs of demographic impact	history archaeology genetics	Suggestive: again, can be multi-causal (famine, long-term climatic shifts, war)
11	iconographic evidence	history archeology	Suggestive: as with new terminology or symptom descriptions, this can be more or less informative; iconographic conventions must always be considered

Table 3.1 lists a range of factors that might usefully be interrogated when asking whether the particular patterns associated with plague's *modus operandi* are at play. These can range from "circumstantial" to "decisive" in giving evidence of plague's presence. Of these eleven types of evidence, Hymes's work on Jin China draws on seven: proximity to contemporary plague-infected regions (now confirmed for Kyrgyzstan by aDNA); surviving Second Plague Pandemic strains in the region; written accounts of both symptoms and swift, large-scale outbreaks; disrupted ruling structures; the adaptation of existing terminology (*geda*) to describe a new disease condition; and the visual (iconographic) comparison of a *geda* to the size of a polo ball, to gauge how big it might be. Archaeological work on this period of northern China's history seems to be minimal, making the imminent retrieval of aDNA as well as other archaeological indicators unlikely. For the time being, then, interrogation of the cultural record for this and other areas of Asia seems to offer the greatest promise of advance.

Opening Our Eyes to an Invisible Past: Time Travel in a Global Middle Ages

In 1898, the Ukrainian epidemiologist Danilo Zabolotny (1866–1929) arrived in the Selenga Valley in northern Mongolia to investigate an ongoing plague outbreak. He reported:

> This is what we have learned. The epidemic has been known here for ten years now under the name of *ven-i, ven-tszay, khai-ven*; this was imported from North-East Mongolia. The Chinese consider the illness as incurable. They distinguish between two forms: the pulmonary form, whose gravest symptom is hemoptysis [spitting blood], and the bubonic form, which is characterised by the appearance of *gada*—the buboes. Entire families perish [of it].[35]

---

35 Zabolotny, "Izcledovanïya po Chumê," 66, as translated and cited by Lynteris, "Jean-Jacques Matignon's Legacy" (2014), 73.

Zabolotny stands just on the cusp of two eras in plague history, when centuries-old traditional understandings of plague were giving way to the new bacteriological ("germ theory") understanding of the disease's causes and mechanisms of spread. In both my article for the inaugural issue of *The Medieval Globe*, "Taking 'Pandemic' Seriously: Making the Black Death Global," and in Hymes's present article, the question of *retrospective diagnosis* looms large.[36] "Retrospective diagnosis" is a term usually used pejoratively by medical historians to refer to naïve or facile attempts to apply modern disease categories to the pre-bacteriological past, in order to positivistically determine what people "must have" experienced, or to assign praise or demerits for the "correctness" of a historical actor's beliefs or actions. aDNA, as a field productive of new historical evidence, is neither naïve nor facile. It has been called a kind of "time travel" that lets modern methods of diagnosis travel back into the past and assess the exact physical conditions that historical actors confronted, just as methods of climate history can retrieve measurements of excessive cold or drought that would have constrained societies of the past.[37] It works from the present backwards, using modern genomes as reference points. Its mantra is: "Everything alive today had ancestors." For the medical historian, the promise of aDNA was never solely about identifying pathogens, as if it was just a matter of sending samples to a diagnostic lab; nor even studying the evolution of the organism for its own sake.[38] As with older attempts at retrospective diagnosis, an emphasis on positivistically identifying the pathogen does not constitute comprehensive disease *history* in and of itself. Disease history entails explaining why that pathogen was present at that given place at that given time *and* how humans responded to the conditions of pain, disability, fear, and death that the pathogen caused.

The early successes of aDNA research were due to taking the testimony of written historical sources seriously and exploring where they told us to look.[39] A technical development in palaeogenetics that came into use in the mid-2010s now allows genetic material to be checked for the presence of plague DNA (and that of other pathogens) even in the absence of documentary or taphonomic indicators that a particular disease might have been present; this was how *S.* Paratyphi C was discovered in twelfth-century Norway and sixteenth-century Mexico. This has led to the extraordinary retrieval of more than a dozen instances of a hitherto unsuspected lineage of plague in Late Neolithic and Bronze Age samples (in places where there are no written records to flag epidemic events), but also to the identification of plague victims in common medieval cemetery sites as well as other,

---

36 Green, "Taking 'Pandemic' Seriously" (2014); Hymes, "Buboes in Thirteenth-Century China" (2022).

37 Krause and Pääbo, "Genetic Time Travel" (2016).

38 It is notable that, among medical historians, nihilistic doubts about the cause of the Black Death (as posited by zoologists, demographers, and economic historians in the late twentieth century) hardly registered at all. See, for example, the acceptance of *Y. pestis* by Dols, *The Black Death* (1977).

39 An exception to these early successes was a sixth-century site in Bavaria, which had not been suspected as holding plague victims yet which yielded positive results in 2003 when an F1 antigen test (a chemical test for a component of plague) was applied; see Little, "Plague Historians" (2011). A decade later, a whole *Y. pestis* genome was retrieved.

more unexpected locations.[40] Clearly, plague's historical impacts have been underestimated on a variety of different fronts. And as noted above, we must assume that plague, in some form or another, existed *somewhere* in Eurasia throughout the medieval period.

However, since plague (because of its virulence) is constantly creating evolutionary deadends by burning through local host populations, we cannot assume that all of its manifold diversity will ever be fully documented. The corollary of the palaeogeneticist's "Everything alive today had ancestors" is "Not everything alive in the past left descendants."[41] A thorough bioarchaeological investigation of Jin-era China or Ayyubid Syria (assuming that Baghdad's history is unrecoverable at this point)[42] would only be decisive if (a) it produced evidence that a pathogen other than *Y. pestis* was involved in the reported thirteenth-century outbreaks or (b) it retrieved *Y. pestis* but of a strain unrelated to the ones involved in the Big Bang. In an *evolutionary* definition of the Second Plague Pandemic, it is not yet possible to confirm the presence of plague in Jin-era China or Ayyubid Iraq or Syria because no confirmatory aDNA has yet been found. But neither has it been looked for.[43]

Since aDNA will always be an exiguous source of evidence, a path forward for medical history is to do what bioarchaeologists do and follow what the *pattern* of evidence is telling us about diseases' paths and effects.[44] The rare retrievals of aDNA (and they will always be rare) are simply nodes in a much larger landscape of evidence that needs to be populated with data from a variety of sources and methods. The more we get clear and unambiguous confirmation of what our historical sources *are already telling us*, the more we should acknowledge that our historical sources are reasonable witnesses to plague's presence. Not perfect: reasonable. Like all historical sources, they demand interrogation, contextualization, and substantiation by other witnesses. The new work postulating the thirteenth-century origins of plague's late-medieval proliferation have taken, not palaeogenetic results, but phylogenetic results as their starting point. They have been grounded not on the happenstance retrieval of isolated, incomplete genomes, but on the growing understanding of plague's overall evolution.

In terms of locating plague, the payoff of employing phylogenetic data historically has been tremendous. The same data that I used to zero in on the marmot-hosted strains of plague in Kyrgyzstan in 2020 is the same data used by Spyrou and colleagues in 2022

---

40 Most recently, see Neumann et al., "Ancient *Yersinia pestis*" (2022); Cessford et al., "Beyond Plague Pits" (2021).

41 A useful summary of how aDNA can and cannot yield evidence of past disease activity is found in Duchêne et al., "Recovery, Interpretation and Use" (2020).

42 Scheiner and Toral, eds., *Baghdād* (2022), especially xiii–xv, itemize several of the reasons why the material remains of medieval Baghdad might never be recovered, e.g., the use of fragile building materials, the numerous conquests of the city, and the limited building activity at certain times, including the Ilkhanate.

43 An opportunity to investigate a burial site in late medieval Cairo was foreclosed because of cultural concerns: see Pradines, "Archaeological Excavations" (2021).

44 An important methodological intervention is offered by Lépinau et al., "Entre peste et famine" (2021), who use the example of the multiple fourteenth-century mass graves at Kutná Hora (Czech Republic) to try, in the absence of aDNA, to differentiate the signs to be expected of mass mortality due to famine vs epidemic disease.

(Plate 3.1, above). Similarly, the dating estimates for the branching events on the *Y. pestis* phylogenetic tree, as supplied by Cui and colleagues and subsequent studies, are what stimulated investigations into Mongol-era Eurasian history. From both China and the Mashriq, we now have the *testimony of physicians* who either describe outbreaks or reported deaths, or who engage in clinical speculation about the nature of a disease characterized by buboes. Obviously, the theoretical systems of medicine familiar to Li Gao and his students differed radically from the Hippocratic–Galenic–Avicennan system that al-Shīrāzī and other Islamicate physicians were operating within. But even in two such contrasting situations, the Chinese physicians and the Islamic ones were clearly struggling to describe and treat comparable physical phenomena.

Crucially, Hymes's present work establishes, not simply that changes in disease description occurred during the thirteenth century, but that medical writers in subsequent centuries continued to respond *as if those changed circumstances persisted.* In other words, what happened in the thirteenth century had permanent effects in terms of the human responses. Already, in 2014, Hymes had assembled a list of major epidemics in southeast China during the century after the Mongol incursions.[45] Without contextualization, we have no way of knowing what caused these, or the many other outbreaks, noted in Chinese annals; or if their extent and severity were "plague-like." However, Hymes makes a very strong argument that the shift in medical thinking that started in the thirteenth century persisted in the centuries thereafter. In Chart 2.2, Hymes assembles references to epidemic *geda* over a nearly six-hundred-year span, from around the fall of the Jin to 1800, divided into fifty-year periods. These data track the longevity of a term; and, of course, word usage can change, as we have noted. Yet when we combine Hymes's analysis with evidence for the evolution of *Yersinia pestis* in Asia, we see that, aside from the continued persistence of a few strains of Bronze Age origin (several of which are no longer lethal to humans),[46] all of the strains of plague currently found in Central and East Asia took their origin in the Big Bang or in the centuries thereafter.[47]

---

45 Specifically, he listed 1331, 1333, 1344, and 1345: Hymes, "Epilogue: A Hypothesis" (2014), 299–300. Others can certainly be identified in Chinese annals.

46 As noted above, since 2015, *Y. pestis* has been detected in a number of Late Neolithic and Bronze Age sites across Eurasia, even though there were no documentary records to indicate its presence. Plague has been postulated as the possible cause of a mass mortality event in late Neolithic Inner Mongolia, about five thousand years ago; see Zhou et al., "The Hamin Mangha Site" (2022).

47 Although genotyping of strains is not yet universal in clinical outbreaks of plague or epidemiological field studies, for those samples that have been characterized in the twentieth and twenty-first century, in northern and western China all reported and genotyped strains fall into either the marmot lineages of the Tian Shan or post-polytomy lineages. He et al., "Distribution and Characteristics" (2021), for example, document the distribution of marmot-caused plague cases in humans for the past sixty years. Comparison with other studies—e.g., Morelli et al., "*Yersinia pestis* Genome Sequencing" (2010); Li et al., "Genetic Source Tracking" (2021), in combination with Feng et al., "Epidemiological Features" (2020); Dai et al., "A Novel Mechanism" (2021); Gao et al., "Human Plague Case" (2021)—shows the following correlations: Inner Mongolia: 2.MED3; Xinjiang: 0.ANT1; Tian Shan: 0.ANT1–3, 0.ANT5; Tibet Plateau: 2.ANT1–2, 2.MED2, 3.ANT1, 1.IN1–2. In northern Mongolia, where Zabolotny was observing a plague outbreak in 1898, 3.ANT2 and 2.ANT3 now dominate. In southern China, strains involved in the Third Plague Pandemic, or their immediate ancestors

Zabolotny's observations of an epidemic disease characterized by *gada* in northern Mongolia in 1898 thus presents us with a link between the medieval terminology and the emerging bacteriological understanding of the late nineteenth century. Just like the continuity of the word-concept *geda*, the strains of *Y. pestis* found in Asia today suggest continuities with *Y. pestis* in the Middle Ages. Zabolotny was himself part of ongoing debate over whether the plague found in northern Mongolia was of local origin or had been imported from southern China, where mapping of the disease had started twenty years earlier.[48] In fact, we can now say with confidence that the strains Zabolotny likely encountered in northern Mongolia had been there for centuries longer than the much younger strains coming out of Yunnan.[49] Whether north or south, nearly all the plague strains found in China would have had a monophyletic origin: they owed their genesis to that single strain of *Y. pestis* that led to the Big Bang. In other words, a single historical circumstance moved one particular strain out of its marmot reservoir in the Tian Shan.

This point merits special emphasis. Genetics itself has established that all outbreaks of plague in Europe, from the 1340s up to the early eighteenth century, were the result of just *one* introduction of plague into western Eurasia.[50] Both the historical record and the phylogenetic profile of surviving *Y. pestis* strains suggest that a long-term, even permanent, plague regime had already become established by the fourteenth century. And since current understandings of plague population biology and ecology dictate that the single introduction of a pathogen into a new environment takes time to amplify—from a single cell that develops the first signature change defining the lineage up to the many billions or trillions of duplications needed to cause disease in millions of new rodents and then human hosts—it stands to reason that the biological processes involved in plague's trans-Eurasian focalizations (most of them invisible or unimportant to humans) would have taken some time to develop.[51] Hymes's proposal of a thirteenth-century origin of the Second Plague Pandemic is compatible with all these considerations.

(1.IN1–3 and 1.ORI), predominate. In western Asia, aside from modern (twentieth-century) introductions of Third Pandemic strains, and tightly localized Bronze Age strains in the Caucasus (0.PE2), all sequenced isolates have been in the 2.MED0–1 and 2.MED4 lineages, which likely did not emerge until the sixteenth century at the earliest, and (aside from 2.MED0) may not have migrated into the western Asia until the late nineteenth or early twentieth century.

48 Lynteris, "Jean-Jacques Mantignon's Legacy" (2014); Hanson, "Visualizing the Geography" (2017).

49 Potentially, samples retrieved from laboratory archives might tell us whether the strain involved in the 1898 outbreak (or in the decades thereafter) was 3.ANT2, a direct product of the Big Bang now found in at least seven of Mongolia's administrative districts; or 2.ANT3, a strain that likely arose from a post-Big Bang reservoir in the early modern period. The strains in the south of China would have been 1.IN3 or 1.ORI, the latter being the cause of the Third Plague Pandemic.

50 On the arguments for Branch 1's introduction into western Eurasia, see Green, "Out of the East" (2022). Jones, *Patterns of Plague* (2022), explores the developing understandings of plague's epidemiological patterns within late medieval and early modern western Europe.

51 No date or locus has yet been proposed for the bifurcation between what would become the 0.ANT3 lineage and what would lead to the Big Bang, the pre-polytomy strain. Since 0.ANT3 remained in the Tian Shan but all the known offspring of the pre-polytomy left the region, save for the Kara-Djigach strain, investigating that divergence will likely produce some answers about precipitating events.

The inaugural issue of *The Medieval Globe* was driven by the question of how historical understandings of the Black Death, and the Second Plague Pandemic more generally, ought to be transformed now that microbiologists had not simply confirmed the causative organism but also the basic outlines of its general evolution. The immediate answer we gave in 2014 was that the pandemic's geography, chronology, and investigative methods all needed to be broadened beyond the parameters used before the genetics turn.[52] Eight years later, the genetic history of *Y. pestis* has continued to develop rapidly, far outpacing work on any other single pathogen. However, decades of still-valuable plague research were done by historians before genetic evidence was available and that work has not yet been integrated into the interpretative historical claims being made by research teams made up exclusively of biologists and archaeologists. For example, the exceptionally comprehensive work by epidemiologist Edward Eckert on the patterns of plague outbreaks in early modern central Europe has been cited only three times in the more than dozen studies published thus far on *Y. pestis* retrieved from that area.[53]

Interdisciplinary synthesis may not be the best way to advance discipline-specific questions, of course, and there are (and will remain) questions that are best addressed within limited analytical frameworks. But to advance the field of plague studies—indeed, to advance the field of global health history generally—there are times when grand syntheses and consilience are needed. One of those times, in the midst of our present pandemic and massive anthropogenic shifts in the Earth's climate, is now.

Defining the Second Plague Pandemic

Grand synthesis and consilience needs to include a reassessment of the stories we tell: the elements of plague stories we take as true without ever questioning them. For centuries, the late medieval "Great Mortality" or "Universal Plague" was defined by *human reports* of catastrophic mortality. As of 2011, that fact in and of itself should have caused plague researchers, whatever their disciplinary background, to stop in their tracks and ask, "Well, if humans across wide geographic expanses are reporting outbreaks among humans, how far back down the biological chain do we have to go to determine *the origin* of this cataclysm?" The economic historian Bruce Campbell, who has invested the most energy in exploring the climatic circumstances that contributed to plague's late medieval re-emergence, envisioned the complicated processes in global weather systems that might have transformed random plague epizootics (localized outbreaks in wild rodent populations) into a pandemic. However, that effort seems to have been premature, because the work of rethinking the chronology of plague's movements across Eurasia had not yet been done.[54]

---

52 Green, "Editor's Introduction" (2014).

53 Eckert, "Boundary Fornation" (1978) and *The Structure of Plagues* (1996).The exceptions are Guellil, "Disease" (2018), Guellil et al., "A Genomic and Historical Synthesis" (2020), and Seguin-Orlando et al., "No Particular Genomic Features" (2021).

54 Campbell, *The Great Transition* (2016); and see observations by Green, "Black as Death" (2018).

Centuries before phylogenetics hinted at an Asian origin of the pandemic (in work published as early as 2004), medieval accounts coming from Mediterranean observers had implicated "the East" in the pandemic. But they proposed no time depth for the pandemic's commencement that extended more than a decade and a half before 1347/48. Nor did any other major thesis that was proposed for the origins of the Black Death before 2013.[55] The new perspectives of Cui and colleagues, Hymes, Green, and Fancy— all claiming a possible thirteenth-century origin for plague's late medieval emergence— are not simply new; they are contrary to nearly seven hundred years of thinking about the Black Death's origins. The weight of historiography that has assumed a shallow time span is the principal reason that the most recent general history of the Black Death—a thousand-page "complete history" by the Norwegian demographic historian Ole Benedictow—insists that the pandemic had its origin in the nearby Caucasus (and not anywhere further east) because, in his survey of the evidence, there was no compelling indication that plague had in fact moved halfway across Eurasia in the decade leading up to 1346.[56]

This understanding that the Black Death had no history prior to the third or fourth decade of the fourteenth century, which has now been taken up by Spyrou and colleagues, is also reinforced by the consistent silence on plague in an increasingly large body of scholarship on the Mongol Empire, the largest land empire in human history. A recent massive volume surveying the field of Mongol studies, for example, published in 2022, makes no mention of any new studies in plague history (including Hymes), repeating instead the traditional chronology of the commencement of the pandemic in the Black Sea region (the 1340s, with passing acknowledgement of the epidemic near Issyk Kul) and citing sources published before the genetics turn.[57] That the largely invisible processes of plague focalization and dissemination should have not been apparent to Mongolists studying the thirteenth century Mongol Empire is not surprising.[58] Partly,

---

55 McNeill, believing that the permanent reservoir of plague was in the Himalayas, proposed that the Mongols had disrupted a plague reservoir there during their incursions into Yunnan during the second half of the thirteenth century. However, he believed that plague stayed within China until it started its westward movement in the 1330s. See Hymes, "Epilogue: A Hypothesis" (2014), 287 and 289n21; Green, "The Four Black Deaths" (2020), 1605.

56 Benedictow, *The Complete History* (2021). Benedictow's views on this point remain unchanged from the original 2004 edition of his book, which appeared before the genetics synthesis.

57 May and Hope, *The Mongol World* (2022), 8–9 and *passim*; Dashdondog's chapter on "Nestorian Christianity" in that volume mentions the *mawtānā* in Semirechye (Kara-Djigach). A rare study that mentions the possibility of plague's presence beyond the oft-cited incident of the siege of Caffa is Shim, "The Postal Roads" (2014), 454–58. Although finding no explicit references to plague in the Chaghadaid khanate (Shim cites only the oft-quoted Aleppan writer Ibn al-Wardī and his fifteenth-century elaborator, the Egyptian historian al-Maqrīzī, neither of whom had direct knowledge of events in the east), Shim nevertheless notes communications and political disruptions between the 1330s and 1350s. Shim assumes a Mongolian origin of the Black Death, which, of course, is contradicted now by genetic data. On Caffa, see Barker, "Laying the Corpses to Rest" (2021).

58 Why the new work on plague's history has not received more attention in Global Middle Ages literature is a separate question. Neither a 2016 special issue on genetics in *Medieval Worlds*, ed. Pohl (*The Genetic Challenge*), nor a special issue of *Past and Present* edited by Holmes and Standen in 2018, nor works published during our own modern pandemic in 2021 and 2022—Heng, *The*

that oversight is because key evidence has only recently been retrieved. al-Shīrāzī's *Akhbār-I Moghūlān* (Mongol News), which recounts the events of the siege of Baghdad and which was instrumental to my realization of a mechanism by which plague may have moved across Central Asia in the thirteenth century, was not rediscovered until 2007, not published in its original Persian until 2010, and not available in a modern translation until 2018. The multiple witnesses to *ṭāʿūn* in thirteenth-century Syria and Egypt were only identified in 2021. And, with the exception of Shim's work on the Mongol postal system, several decades of intense study on the Chaghadaid realm has produced not even a hint that plague might have been periodically erupting out of its Tian Shan habitats.[59]

It is not surprising, therefore, that the team studying the Kara-Djigach site in Kyrgyzstan should have come to their work assuming that the "pestilence" afflicting the Nestorian community in the late 1330s was not simply caused by *Yersinia pestis* (as, in fact, they were able to confirm), but that this Central Asian outbreak should be directly linked in a tight causal chain to the oft-told account of plague's spread from Caffa on the Black Sea in the 1340s. The claim of such a rapid spread out of Central Asia has been floated in plague studies since the 1950s, and this research team's work, ever since 2011, has been premised on an assumption that the traditional narrative of plague's single-point entry into Europe in 1347 was true—as was the very short timeframe for the beginning phases of the Second Plague Pandemic.[60] It is clear that new analytical modes will have to be developed to piece together evidence of landscape disruptions that would have accompanied epizootic spread of plague.[61] As with the later medieval climate shifts,[62] so, too, is it necessary to investigate biological shifts that had previously been beyond both contemporaries' and modern historians' ken.

In examining the geography involved, the language used, the rhetorical structures employed, the social networks and political goals that may have been operative at the

---

Global Middle Ages (2021); Brubaker et al., eds., *Global Byzantium* (2022)—address how either plague or any other hemispherically- or globally-disseminated disease should be incorporated into the field's remit. Borgolte, *Die Welten des Mittelalters* (2022), a thousand-page synthesis, includes only passing mentions of the Black Death and relies on pre-genetics literature; on China in particular he asserts that it did not experience plague until the seventeenth century (905n501). Two welcome exceptions are Sarris, "Climate and Disease" (2020), which incorporates the latest work on plague in late antiquity; and Heng, *Teaching the Global Middle Ages* (2022), a pedagogical handbook which acknowledges the new "global" history of leprosy as reconstructed from genetics. On trans-Eurasian approaches to medieval medical history, see Yoeli-Tlalim, *ReOrienting Histories* (2021).

59 The most recent survey on Chaghadaid historiography is Jackson, "Mongols of Central Asia" (2018), which never mentions plague. Shim was under the belief that plague emerged out of Mongolia, when in fact the cumulative evidence from genetics is that the new, highly virulent strains of plague of the late Middle Ages were taken *to* Mongolia: see note 47 above.

60 Green, "Out of the East" (2022), drawing on phylogenetic indications and documentary records, raises several questions about whether the standard narrative of a single point of entry of plague into mid-fourteenth-century Europe is supportable.

61 Evidence for massive landscape disruptions in Song-era China is being collected; see Chen, "Kaifeng" (2021).

62 Pfister and Wanner, *Climate and Society* (2021).

time, Hymes's trilogy of studies reconstructing these episodes in Jin China has laid the foundation for a history of plague in China that extends up to the present day. As more genomes of *Y. pestis* become available (whether "ancient" or modern), it will become increasingly possible to establish the ages of different plague reservoirs, which in turn enhance our ability to link them to historical outbreaks.[63] What Hymes has done for Jin China might potentially be done for other areas of Asia, assuming that clusters of suitable sources fortuitously survive. In some cases, investigations will yield only ambiguity. The work that Arabist Claudia Maria Tresso has done in documenting Ibn Baṭṭūṭa's (d. 1368/9) precise rhetorical and semantic nuances in describing disease landscapes in both India and the western Asia suggests that there are crucial differences in the "diagnostic value" of disease references coming from trained physicians like Li Gao or al-Shīrāzī and a layman like Ibn Baṭṭūṭa. The latter uses the medically specific term *ṭā'ūn* (meaning both the disease plague and the diagnostic symptom, the bubo) exactly once in the entire text of his *Riḥla* or "Travels," even during the two years when he is passing through the highly active plague landscape of western Asia and North Africa upon his return from twenty-three years of travelling through South and East Asia. In all other instances—whether talking about epidemics in India or the Middle East—he uses only the generic *wabā'* ("epidemic"). And yet a mass of contextual evidence makes us confident that *Yersinia pestis* was indeed circulating in western Eurasia upon his return during those years, even though no aDNA of the bacterium has yet been retrieved from the eastern or southern shores of the Mediterranean. Meanwhile, for the Indian subcontinent, there is neither palaeogenetic nor phylogenetic evidence, nor substantial enough documentary evidence, to discern what disease(s) might have been involved in the several episodes of *wabā'* Ibn Baṭṭūṭa describes there. That India would *later* experience plague, we can be confident; but that is the sort of careful attention to chronology that is now so vital to advancing work in this field.[64]

Importantly, Tresso has also established how much systematic work will be needed to root mistaken assumptions out of disease histories, some of which go back through generations of scholarship. In the case of Ibn Baṭṭūṭa's experiences in India, Tresso finds a long trail of "diagnoses" based on the choices modern translators and editors made in translating *wabā'*: some writing before, some after the impact of the new bacteriology of the later nineteenth century.[65] The efforts of Hymes and Tresso thus show us the

63 For example, Hanson, "Late Imperial Epidemiology" (2022), engages in an extended and important analysis to determine whether major epidemics in early modern China were plague or smallpox. Whereas smallpox (as we understand it now) has no fixed reservoir but was constantly moving through different human populations while plague can often be tied to fixed, long-term environmental foci, an evolutionary approach holds the promise of helping to track specific plague strains through their historical landscapes. For genotyping and geolocation information currently available, see note 47 above.

64 Tresso, "A Two-Year Journey" (2021) and "India's Epidemics" (forthcoming).

65 Two deeply rooted errors arose out of interpretations of the Arabic word *wabā'*, whose default meaning is simply "epidemic." Some translators rendered it as plague (*peste*, *Pest*, etc.), others as "cholera." The latter misinterpretation is in fact found in many historical studies from the nineteenth century on, when *wabā'* was applied to the newly pandemic disease of cholera (what we

standard of philological mastery, exacting attention to chronology and the constraints of genre, plus awareness of a range of biological possibilities, that need to go into a new kind of informed disease history. William McGrath has now started similar work on the medieval history of Tibet.[66]

Collectively, these works mark a turning point in what historical research is able to do if it abandons simplistic "diagnoses" based on words (or images) alone and instead insists on deeply contextualized interrogations that combine multiple indicators. The new evolutionary paradigm of plague history—built upon the combined approaches of phylogenetics and palaeogenetics—has given us a surprisingly consistent outline of plague history over five millennia. Filling in the millions of missing stories that this extraordinarily lethal pathogen carved out across the landscapes of Afro-Eurasia (and later the Americas) remains the central task of disease history. Whether we call our approaches *emic/etic* or natural-realist/historical-conceptual, this field is moving toward embracing the fact that the reconstruction of a biological past is now possible in a way that does not depend solely on the necessarily blinkered vision of historical actors. But historical human actors can also tell us more than we sometimes expect. Hymes's exacting reconstruction of the experiences and observations of Li Gao and his contemporaries in thirteenth-century Jin China sets a standard to which the entire field of plague studies should aspire. And it throws down a challenge before the developing fields of both global medieval studies and Global Health History: in our own new age of pandemics, is it not now time to wrestle squarely with the ways pre-modern globalizing forces were themselves the mechanisms by which local outbreaks turned into pandemics?

A century ago, the Malayan plague epidemiologist, Wu Liande, envisioned a map of plague that saw the marmot colonies of the Tian Shan as an epicentre from which plague likely spread both east and west during the later Middle Ages.[67] But like all plague researchers up until the second decade of the twenty-first century, he had no means to establish any chronological specificity for the epidemiological landscape he envisioned. We do. Asia can no longer be left off this map, and it is a map that historians, first and foremost, must draft.

---

understand now to be the disease caused by *Vibrio cholerae*).

66 McGrath, "The Princess and the Plague" (2021) and "The *Vase of Ambrosia*" (2021).

67 Wu, "The Original Home of Plague" (1924). (Wu used the transcription "Lien-teh" in his publications; "Liande" is the modern form.) Wu was writing before biochemical assays were developed to differentiate among "biovars" of *Yersinia pestis*. His essay merits revisiting as a snapshot of the state of historical plague thinking at the time, which was actually in the second generation of bacteriological approaches to reconstructing plague's history in East Asia. On earlier work on plague in the marmots of Mongolia and Manchuria, see Lynteris, "Jean-Jacques Mantignon's Legacy" (2014); on earlier maps of plague in China (which were also the first maps of any infectious disease there), see Hanson, "Visualizing the Geography" (2017), 228–32.

Bibliography

Barker, Hannah. "Laying the Corpses to Rest: Grain, Embargoes, and *Yersinia pestis* in the Black Sea, 1346–1348." *Speculum* 96, no. 1 (January 2021): 97–126.

Benedictow, Ole. *The Complete History of the Black Death*. Rev. ed. Woodbridge: Boydell, 2021.

Borgolte, Michael. *Die Welten des Mittelalters: Globalgeschichte eines Jahrtausends*. Munich: Beck, 2022.

Bos, Kirsten I. et al. "A Draft Genome of *Yersinia pestis* from Victims of the Black Death." *Nature* 478 (2011): 506–10.

Brubaker, Leslie et al., eds. *Global Byzantium: Papers from the Fiftieth Spring Symposium of Byzantine Studies*. London: Routledge, 2022.

Buikstra, Jane E. et al. "Introduction: Scientific Rigor in Paleopathology." *International Journal of Paleopathology* 19 (2017): 80–87.

Campbell, Bruce. *The Great Transition: Climate, Disease and Society in the Late Medieval World*. Cambridge: Cambridge University Press, 2016.

Cessford, Craig et al.. "Beyond Plague Pits: Using Genetics to Identify Responses to Plague in Medieval Cambridgeshire." *European Journal of Archaeology* 24, no. 4 (November 2021): 496–518.

Chen, Yuan. "Kaifeng: What it Took to Feed, Furnish, and Fortify the World's Largest City, 960–1127." Lecture presented to the John Hope Franklin Center at Duke University, November 17, 2021: YouTube video, https://www.youtube.com/watch?v=-iAzaOeFKxo, accessed August 12, 2022.

Cui, Yujun et al.. "Historical Variations in Mutation Rate in an Epidemic Pathogen, *Yersinia pestis*." *PNAS* 110, no. 2 (2013): 577–82.

Dai, Ruixia et al. "A Novel Mechanism of Streptomycin Resistance *in Yersinia pestis*: Mutation in the rpsL Gene." *PLoS Neglected Tropical Diseases* 15, no. 4 (2021): e0009324.

Dashdondog, Bayarsaikhan. "Nestorian Christianity among the Mongols." In *The Mongol World,* edited by Timothy May and Michael Hope, 631–41. New York: Taylor and Francis, 2022.

Dols, Michael. *The Black Death in the Middle East*. Princeton: Princeton University Press, 1977.

Duchêne, Sebastián et al. "The Recovery, Interpretation and Use of Ancient Pathogen Genomes." *Current Biology* 30 (October 5, 2020), R1215–R1231.

Eckert, Edward A. "Boundary Formation and Diffusion of Plague: Swiss Epidemics from 1562 to 1669." *Annales de Démographie Historique* for 1978 (1978): 49–80.

____ . *The Structure of Plagues and Pestilences in Early Modern Europe. Central Europe 1560–1640*. Basel: Karger, 1996.

Ellenblum, Ronnie. *The Collapse of the Eastern Mediterranean: Climate Change and the Decline of the East, 950–1072 AD*. Cambridge: Cambridge University Press, 2012.

Fancy, Nahyan. "Knowing the Signs of Disease: Plague in the Arabic Medical Commentaries between the First and Second Pandemics." In *Death and Disease in the Medieval and Early Modern World*, edited by Lori Jones and Nükhet Varlık, 35–66. York: York University Press, 2022.

Fancy, Nahyan and Monica H. Green, "Plague and the Fall of Baghdad (1258)," *Medical History* 65, no. 2 (April 2021): 157–77.

Feng, Yilan et al. "Epidemiological Features of Four Human Plague Cases in the Inner Mongolia Autonomous Region, China in 2019." *Biosafety and Health* 2 (2020): 44–48.

Gao, Jianwei et al. "Human Plague Case Diagnosed in Ningxia Tracked to Animal Reservoirs— Inner Mongolia Autonomous Region, China, 2021," *China CDC Weekly* 3, no. 2 (December 24, 2021): 1109–12.

Grauer, Anne. "A Century of Paleopathology." Special Centennial Anniversary Issue. *American Journal of Physical Anthropology* [now *American Journal of Biological Anthropology*] 165, no. 4 (April 2018): 904–14.

Green, Monica H. "Black as Death," essay review of *The Great Transition: Climate, Disease and Society in the Late-Medieval World*, by Bruce Campbell (2016). *Inference: International Review of Science* 4, no. 1 (June 1, 2018): http://inference-review.com/article/black-as-death.

——. "Editor's Introduction" to *The Medieval Globe* 1 (2014): 9–26. Reprinted as *Pandemic Disease in the Medieval World: Rethinking the Black Death*, edited by Monica H. Green, with Carol Symes. Bradford and Kalamazoo: Arc Medieval [Humanities] Press, 2015.

——. "The Four Black Deaths." *American Historical Review* 125, no. 5 (December 2020): 1600–31, plus Supplemental Material, "Marmots and Their Plague Strains," https://doi.org/10.1093/ahr/rhaa511.

——. "The Great Dying: The Epidemiological and Medical Implications of Old and New World Encounters in the Pre- and Post-Contact Eras." In *History in the Time of Pandemics: Essays and Bibliographies*, edited by Stephen P. Weldon and Neeraja Sankaran. IsisCB Special Issue, n.p.: Isis, 2021: https://drive.google.com/file/d/1wYlHpY5l11HE5Vk2qwvxYSeiX KqEZQSo/view, accessed August 15, 2022.

——. "Out of the East (and West and South): A Response to Philip Slavin." *Past and Present* 256, no. 1 (August 2022): 283–323.

——. "Putting Africa on the Black Death Map: Narratives from Genetics and History." *Afriques* 9 (December 24, 2018): http://journals.openedition.org/afriques/2125.

——. "Taking 'Pandemic' Seriously: Making the Black Death Global." *The Medieval Globe* 1 (2014): 27–61. Reprinted as *Pandemic Disease in the Medieval World: Rethinking the Black Death*, edited by Monica H. Green, with Carol Symes. Bradford and Kalamazoo: Arc Medieval [Humanities] Press, 2015.

——. "When Numbers Don't Count: Changing Perspectives on the Justinianic Plague." *Eidolon* (November 18, 2019): https://eidolon.pub/when-numbers-dont-count-56a2b3c3d07, accessed August 20, 2022.

Green, Monica H., with Carol Symes, eds. *The Medieval Globe* 1 (2014). Reprinted as *Pandemic Disease in the Medieval World: Rethinking the Black Death*, edited by Monica H. Green, with Carol Symes. Bradford and Kalamazoo: Arc Medieval [Humanities] Press, 2015: http://scholarworks.wmich.edu/medieval_globe/1.

Guellil, Meriam. "Disease during the Second Plague Pandemic (14th–18th Century CE): Genomic, Metagenomic and Phylogenetic Analysis of ancient DNA from Putative Plague Victims." PhD diss., University of Oslo, 2018.

Guellil, Meriam et al. "A Genomic and Historical Synthesis of Plague in 18th-Century Eurasia." *PNAS* 117, no. 45 (October 26, 2020): 28328–35.

Haller, Magdalena et al. "Mass Burial Genomics Reveals Outbreak of Enteric Paratyphoid Fever in the Late Medieval Trade City Lübeck." *iScience* 24, no. 5 (May 21, 2021): 102419.

Hanson, Marta E. "Late Imperial Epidemiology, Part 2: New Material and Conceptual Methods from the 1980s to 2010s." In *The Routledge Handbook of Chinese Medicine*, edited by Vivienne Lo and Michael Stanley-Baker, 245–81. London: Routledge, 2022.

——. "Visualizing the Geography of the Diseases of China: Western Disease Maps from Analytical Tools to Tools of Empire, Sovereignty, and Public Health Propaganda, 1878–1929." *Science in Context* 30 (2017): 219–80.

He, Zhaokai et al. "Distribution and Characteristics of Human Plague Cases and *Yersinia pestis* Isolates from 4 *Marmota* Plague Foci, China, 1950–2019." *Emerging Infectious Diseases* 27, no. 10 (October 2021): 2544–53.

Heng, Geraldine. *The Global Middle Ages: An Introduction*. Cambridge: Cambridge University Press, 2021.

Heng, Geraldine, ed. *Teaching the Global Middle Ages*. MLA Options for Teaching. New York: Modern Languages Association of America, 2022.

Holmes, Catherine, and Naomi Standon, eds. "The Global Middle Ages." Special issue, *Past and Present* 238, Supplement 13 (2018).

Hughes, Jennifer Scheper. *The Church of the Dead: The Epidemic of 1576 and the Birth of Christianity in the Americas*. New York: New York University Press, 2021.

Hymes, Robert. "Buboes in Thirteenth-Century China: Evidence from Chinese Medical Writings," *The Medieval Globe* 8, no. 1 (2022): 3–59.

———. "Epilogue: A Hypothesis on the East Asian Beginnings of the *Yersinia pestis* Polytomy." *The Medieval Globe* 1 (2014): 285–308. Reprinted as *Pandemic Disease in the Medieval World: Rethinking the Black Death*, edited by Monica H. Green, with Carol Symes. Bradford and Kalamazoo: Arc Medieval [Humanities] Press, 2015.

———. "A Tale of Two Sieges: Liu Qi, Li Gao, and Epidemics in the Jin-Yuan Transition," *Journal of Song-Yuan Studies* 50 (2021): 295–363. Includes as a separate downloadable appendix, "Patients and Associates of Li Gao, and Their Associations."

Jackson, Peter. "The Mongols of Central Asia and the Qara'unas." *Iran* 56, no. 1 (2018): 91–103.

Jones, Lori. *Patterns of Plague: Changing Ideas about Plague in England and France, 1348–1750*. Montréal and Kingston: Queen's University Press, 2022.

Krause, Johannes, and Svante Pääbo. "Genetic Time Travel." *Genetics* 203, no. 1 (May 1, 2016): 9–12.

Lépinau, Auxane de et al. "Entre peste et famine: caractérisation d'une crise de mortalité par l'étude de trois sépultures multiples du site de Kutná Hora – Sedlec (République tchèque, XIVe siècle) / Between Plague and Famine: Characterization of a Mortality Crisis Through the Study of Three Mass Graves from the Kutná Hora – Sedlec Site (Czech Republic, 14th Century)." *Bulletins et mémoires de la Société d'Anthropologie de Paris* 32, no. 2 (2021): https://doi.org/10.4000/bmsap.7664.

Li, Jianyun et al. "Genetic Source Tracking of Human Plague Cases in Inner Mongolia-Beijing, 2019." *PLOS Neglected Tropical Diseases* 15, no. 8 (2021): e0009558.

Little, Lester K. "Plague Historians in Lab Coats." *Past and Present* 213 (2011): 267–90.

Lynteris, Christos. "Jean-Jacques Matignon's Legacy on Russian Plague Research in North-East China and Inner Asia (1898–1910)." *Extrême-Orient, Extrême-Occident* 37 (2014): 61–89.

McGrath, William A. "The Princess and the Plague: Explaining Epidemics in Imperial Tibet, Khotan, and Central Asia." *Journal of the American Oriental Society* 141 (2021): 637–60.

———. "The *Vase of Ambrosia*: A Scriptural Cycle about the Black Death in Tibet." In "Asian Medicine and COVID-19," ed. Michael Stanley-Baker, Ronit Yoeli-Tlalim, and Dolly Yang, 214–29. Special Issue: *Asian Medicine* 16 (2021).

Marien, Gisele. "The Black Death in Early Ottoman Territories: 1347–1550." Master's thesis, Bilkent University, 2009.

May, Timothy and Michael Hope, eds. *The Mongol World*. New York: Taylor and Francis, 2022.

Morelli, Giovanna et al. "*Yersinia pestis* Genome Sequencing Identifies Patterns of Global Phylogenetic Diversity." *Nature Genetics* 42, no. 12 (2010): 1140–45.

Neumann, Gunnar U. et al. "Ancient *Yersinia pestis* and *Salmonella enterica* Genomes from Bronze Age Crete." *Current Biology* 32, no. 16 (August 22, 2022): 3641–49.e8.

Pfister, Christian and Heinz Wanner. *Climate and Society in Europe—The Last Thousand Years*. Bern: Haupt, 2021.

Pohl, Walter, ed. "The Genetic Challenge to Medieval History and Archaeology." Special Issue, *Medieval Worlds* 4 (2016).

Pradines, Stéphane. "Archaeological Excavations of Bāb al-Ghurayb Cemetery: Plague Epidemics and the Ruin of Fourteenth-Century Cairo." *Mamlūk Studies Review* 24 (2021): 117–68.

Sarris, Peter. "Climate and Disease." In *A Companion to the Global Early Middle Ages*, edited by Erik Hermans, 511–37. Leeds: Arc Humanities Press, 2020.

———. "New Approaches to the 'Plague of Justinian'." *Past and Present* 254, no. 1 (February 2022): 315–46.

Scheiner, Jens, and Isabel Toral, eds. *Baghdād: From Its Beginnings to the 14th Century*. Leiden: Brill, 2022.

Seguin-Orlando, Andaine et al. "No Particular Genomic Features Underpin the Dramatic Economic Consequences of 17th Century Plague Epidemics in Italy," *iScience* 24, no. 4 (April 23, 2021): 102383.

Shim, Hosung. "The Postal Roads of the Great Khans in Central Asia under the Mongol-Yuan Empire." *Journal of Song-Yuan Studies* 44 (2014): 405–69.

Spyrou, Maria A. et al. "The Source of the Black Death in Fourteenth-Century Central Eurasia." *Nature* 606 (June 15, 2022): 718–24.

Tang, Deming et al. "Plague Outbreak of a *Marmota himalayana* Family Emerging from Hibernation." *Vector-Borne and Zoonotic Diseases* 22, no. 8 (August 9, 2022): 410–18.

Tresso, Claudia Maria. "India's Epidemics in the *Riḥla* of Ibn Baṭṭūṭa: Plague, Cholera or Lexical Muddle?" *Bulletin of the School of Oriental and African Studies*, forthcoming.

———. "A Two-year Journey under the Arrows of the Black Death: The Medieval Plague Pandemic in Ibn Baṭṭūṭa's *Travels*." *Journal of Arabic and Islamic Studies* 21 (2021): 137–89.

Vågene, Åshild J. et al. "*Salmonella enterica* Genomes from Victims of a Major Sixteenth-Century Epidemic in Mexico." *Nature Ecology & Evolution* 2 (2018): 520–28.

Varlık, Nükhet. *Plague and Empire in the Early Modern Mediterranean World: The Ottoman Experience, 1347–1600*. Cambridge: Cambridge University Press, 2015.

———. "Plague in the Mediterranean/Islamicate World: A Bibliographic Review. Version 3." In *History in the Time of Pandemics: Essays and Bibliographies*, edited by Stephen P. Weldon and Neeraja Sankaran. IsisCB Special Issue, n.p.: Isis, 2021: https://isiscb.org/special-issue-on-pandemics/essay.html?essayID=11, accessed August 26, 2022.

Wu, Lien-Teh. "The Original Home of Plague." In *Far Eastern Association of Tropical Medicine, Transactions of the Fifth Biennial Congress Held at Singapore, 1923*, edited by A. L. Hoops and J. W. Scharff, 286–304. London: Bale & Danielsson, 1924.

Xi, Jinxiao et al. "First Case Report of Human Plague Caused by Excavation, Skinning, and Eating of a Hibernating Marmot (*Marmota himalayana*)." *Frontiers in Public Health* 10 (2022): 910872.

Yoeli-Tlalim, Ronit. *ReOrienting Histories of Medicine: Encounters along the Silk Roads*. London: Bloomsbury, 2021.

Zabolotny, Danilo K. "Izcledovanïya po Chumê; Stat'ya Pervaya" [Research on Plague; First Article]. *Arkhiv Biologicheskikh Nauk* 8, no. 1 (1901): 59–77.

Zhou, Yawei et al. "The Hamin Mangha Site: Mass Deaths and Abandonment of a Late Neolithic Settlement in Northeastern China." *Asian Perspectives* 61, no. 1 (2022): 28–49.

Monica H. Green (monica.h.green@gmail.com) is a historian of medicine specializing in the history of premodern Europe and the comparative history of global health. Trained in the History of Science at Princeton University, she has taught and held fellowships at leading institutions such as Duke University; the Institute for Advanced Study; and All Souls College, Oxford. Both her research and her teaching have been honoured by top prizes, and she was recently recognized by having a research prize named in her honour by the Medieval Academy of America, of which she is an elected Fellow. Her earlier works include an edition and translation of the compendium of writings on women's healthcare known as the *Trotula* (2001), and an examination of the role of gender in the formation of the field of gynecology, *Making Women's Medicine Masculine* (2008). In addition to on-going work on the impact of Arabic medicine in Europe in the eleventh and twelfth centuries, she is currently completing *The Black Death: A Global History*, which melds new insights from genetics with a reinterrogation of the documentary record of the world's most devastating pandemic.

Abstract In the eight years since the inaugural issue of *The Medieval Globe* appeared in 2014, studies of the Second Plague Pandemic have proliferated. Yet Asia's history has lagged somewhat behind in this renewed drive to make sense of plague's late medieval and early modern diffusion, including what is widely considered the most devastating pandemic episode in human history, the Black Death. That omission is unlikely to continue: the latest work by Robert Hymes, appearing in this issue, furthers his original 2014 argument (followed by a 2021 supplement) that, as early as the thirteenth century, Chinese physicians were struggling to understand what seems to have been a new disease characterized by pronounced swellings (buboes or *geda*) and swift mortality. Coincidentally, new work in palaeogenetics has confirmed that a proliferation of plague did indeed occur in medieval Central Asia. But Hymes's work, based on traditional modes of textual analysis, is at odds with the chronology proposed by palaeogeneticists working from archaeological and genetic data and computerized reconstructions of the evolutionary history of *Yersinia pestis*, which suggest that plague's explosive profusion did not happen until the fourteenth century. With more than a century's discrepancy in their timing of plague's re-emergence, these two approaches have complicated Asia's history once again. Here, I argue that a global approach that examines the larger connectivities of late medieval Eurasia and (in this case) that takes the possibilities of a unified "biological archive" seriously, may provide a path out of the impasse and help to integrate disease history more squarely into the topical and methodological remit of global history and the Global History of Health.

Keywords medical history, retrospective diagnosis, global health, pathogen evolution, Mongol Empire, Second Plague Pandemic, Black Death, palaeogenetics